MEMORY BANK FOR CHEMOTHERAPY

Jones and Bartlett Series in Oncology

MEMORY BANK FOR CHEMOTHERAPY

Third Edition

Fredrica A. Preston, RNC, NP, AOCN

Oncology Nurse Practitioner
North Shore Cancer Center
Peabody, Massachusetts

Cecilia Wilfinger, RN, BS, CIC

Nurse Epidemiologist
Northwest Covenant Medical Center
Dover, New Jersey

Jones and Bartlett Publishers

Sudbury, Massachusetts

Boston   London   Singapore

Editorial, Sales, and Customer Service Offices
Jones and Bartlett Publishers
40 Tall Pine Drive
Sudbury, MA 01776
(508) 443-5000/(800) 832-0034
info@jbpub.com
http://www.jbpub.com

Jones and Bartlett Publishers International
Barb House, Barb Mews
London W6 7PA
UK

Library of Congress Cataloging-in-Publication Data
Preston, Fredrica A.
    Memory bank for chemotherapy / Fredrica A. Preston, Cecilia
Wilfinger. — 3rd ed.
        p.   cm.
    Includes bibliographical references.
    ISBN 0-86720-740-X
    1. Cancer—Chemotherapy—Congresses. 2. Antineoplastic agents
—Congresses. 3. Cancer—Nursing—Congresses. I. Wilfinger,
Cecilia. II. Title.
    [DNLM: 1. Oncologic Nursing—handbooks. 2. Neoplasms—drug
therapy—handbooks. 3. Antineoplastic Agents—therapeutic use
—nurses' instruction.   WY 49 P937m 1997]
RC271.C5P73   1997
616.99'4061—dc20
DNLM/DLC
for Library of Congress   96-21045
                                                                CIP

Printed in the United States of America
00 99 98 97 96   10 9 8 7 6 5 4 3 2 1

Contents

Preface

As recently as twenty-five years ago, chemotherapy was viewed with skepticism among both health care providers and patients. Its efficacy was a source of controversy, its utilization was limited to a very select group of cancers, and its side effects were poorly managed because of a lack of knowledge and resources. Usually, the administration of these drugs was the province of the physician, and the nurse's role was limited to providing comfort measures to the patients suffering from the treatment's side effects. Today, after many clinical trials and much research, chemotherapy has achieved the status of primary modality in the treatment of several cancers.

Nurses have played an important role in this evolution of chemotherapy. Most chemotherapy is administered by nurses now, and nurses have developed interventions to minimize the physical and emotional consequence of treatment-related side effects. Oncology nurses have assumed the major responsibility for the development, utilization, and evaluation of patient education materials. They have assumed an active role in clinical trials as data managers, protocol nurses, and investigators. Through the efforts of nursing research, quality of life studies are accepted companion studies to chemotherapy research protocols. Nurses have also assumed numerous administrative responsibilities in cancer care, such as managing oncology settings, developing standards of practice, and maintaining fiscal integrity without compromising the quality of care.

Nurses provide care for chemotherapy patients in the inpatient, clinic, office, or home setting. To assure quality and consistency across settings, adherence to the same standards of practice is enforced. This manual is designed as an easily readable pocket reference for chemotherapy administration, identification and management of side effects, and education of patients receiving chemotherapy. Background information on the cell cycle and its relevance to chemotherapy is included. Patient assessment guides and two quick drug administration checklists are provided.

Deliverance of high-quality health care is a constant challenge to the nurse caring for the patient with cancer. We hope this pocket reference will be a valuable reference for nurses who meet this challenge in their daily practice.

Foreword

With changes in the delivery of health care, persons
with cancer and their families, as well as nurses, face
new challenges in coping with the effects of cancer
treatment. Intensive treatments, previously administered in inpatient settings, are now administered to
outpatients, with patients and family members re-
sponsible for follow-up care. Inpatient protocols are
constantly changing, with the emphasis being on
immediate and long-term patient outcomes. Nurses
working with persons receiving chemotherapy must
constantly apply a wide range of knowledge about the
actions of the drugs, techniques of administration, and
side effects. The increasing need for nurses with spe-
cialized knowledge in cancer treatment creates a need
for ongoing education.

Memory Bank for Chemotherapy, Third Edition, is a
comprehensive manual that presents the information
nurses must have to participate in the administration
of therapy and care of patients. The information is
organized to facilitate quick and easy reference.

The authors bring a unique blend of knowledge
and expertise to the project of assimilating this vast
body of knowledge in a concise text. Cecilia Wilfinger
has worked extensively in the past as an administra-
tor and as an oncology nurse specialist in a large
practice of cancer patients. She has served as an educational consultant, teaching home care nurses about
chemotherapy.

Fredrica Preston has had much input into the estab-
lishment of educational programs and guidelines for
oncology nursing practice. She has served as clinical
associate faculty of the Hunter-Bellevue School of
Nursing, Graduate Division, and currently works as an
oncology nurse practitioner.

Their varied backgrounds are reflected in the text,
which captures the sensitivity and knowledge that can
only be gained through years of clinical experience. By
translating their experience into a comprehensive
reference, the authors are making a great contribution
to the cancer nursing literature.

Patricia E. Green, RN, MSN, FAAN
National Vice President for Patient Care Services
American Cancer Society

Acknowledgments

We would like to thank Jean Jenkins, RN, MS, and
Terry Mass, RN, MSN, who took time out of their very
busy personal and professional lives to review this
manuscript. We are indebted to William Lew Quan,
Pharm.D, of the University of California, Los Angeles,
Bowyer Multidisciplinary Oncology Clinic, for a
thoughtful and comprehensive review of the chemotherapeutic drugs presented. We would also like to
thank Rose Mary Carroll-Johnson, RN, MN, whose
faith and constant encouragement were major factors
in the publication of this book.

I

Overview of Chemotherapy

The use of drugs to cure or control cancer is relatively new in comparison to the use of surgery and radiation. This form of treatment began around 1942 as a result of an accident with nitrogen mustard gas, which was being studied for possible military use. The individuals exposed to this gas were found to have low white cell counts. Some early researchers felt that if this gas caused the decrease in WBCs, then it had potential for lowering high WBCs in patients with leukemia.

The first patient to receive such a treatment did have a response to the drug though this response was brief. This experiment was the birth of the collaborative research efforts we see today. Almost half a century later, a concerted, organized effort in the treatment of cancer with chemotherapeutic agents continues.

Cell Cycle

Most chemotherapy drugs act by affecting cellular enzymes. These enzymes are involved in DNA synthesis and/or function. DNA synthesis occurs only when cells are processing through the cell cycle.

The cell cycle refers to five phases of growth and development all cells, normal and neoplastic, go through during their life cycle (see fig. 1.1). Specific growth and development activities occur during each of these phases.

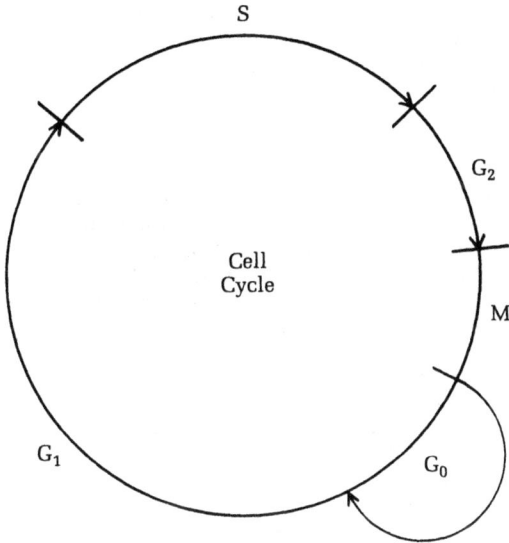

Phases of the cell cycle:
S   = DNA synthesis
G_2 = The gap between DNA synthesis and mitosis;
     active RNA and protein synthesis
M   = Mitosis
G_0 = Resting phase
G_1 = The gap between mitosis and DNA synthesis;
     active RNA and protein synthesis

Figure 1.1.   Cell cycle.

Chemotherapy drugs interfere with the cellular activities during one or more of these phases.

Cell cycle specific (CCS) drugs affect cellular activity during specific phases of the cell cycle excluding the G_0 or resting phase. An example of a CCS drug is methotrexate, which affects the cell during the S phase by inhibiting DNA synthesis. Cell cycle nonspecific (CCNS) drugs can affect the cell during any phase, including the resting phase. Actively dividing cells are far more sensitive to the effects of chemotherapy than nondividing cells. An example of a CCNS drug is cyclophosphamide. The phases of the cell cycle are:

G_0: Resting phase—all cellular activities continue except reproduction; least sensitive to chemotherapy (indefinite time period)

G_1: RNA and protein synthesis (several hours to days)

S: DNA synthesis (10–20 hours)

G_2: RNA and protein synthesis (2–10 hours)

M: Mitosis phase, cell division (30–60 minutes)

Chemotherapy drugs can be further divided based on their structure and function during the cell cycle.

Alkylating Agents

CCNS

Damage the completed DNA molecule

Antimetabolites

CCS during the S phase
Inhibit protein synthesis
Incorrectly substitute for the metabolite
   needed for DNA synthesis making cellular
   reproduction impossible

Nitrosoureas

CCNS
Inhibit DNA and RNA synthesis
Lipid soluble for CNS access allowing them to
   cross the blood brain barrier

Antitumor Antibiotics

CCNS and CCS during the G_2 and M phases
Interfere with cell division and transcription
   of RNA

Mitotic Inhibitors

CCS during the M phase
Interfere with mitotic spindle formation,
   thereby preventing cellular division
Interfere with protein and nucleic acid
   formation

Miscellaneous Drugs

Action unknown or poorly understood

Occasionally, single agent chemotherapy will be
the treatment of choice for a particular cancer.
An example of this would be the use of chlorambucil for the treatment of chronic lymphocytic

leukemia. While single agent chemotherapy is employed, the combination of two or more agents have clearly achieved therapeutic advantage and expanded the use of chemotherapy. Malignant cells are not of uniform composition within a given tumor. If these tumor cells were all alike, then a single agent would be adequate for all types of cancer. Cells within the tumor are in different stages of growth and development. Since different classes of chemotherapy affect the cells at different stages, combination chemotherapy has a greater chance of destroying a larger number of cancer cells.

There are several important factors to consider when choosing a combination of chemotherapeutic drugs:

1. Select drugs that as single agents are known to have an effect on the type of tumor cells.
2. Select drugs that act at different stages of the cell cycle.
3. Select drugs whose major toxicities affect different body systems. Remember that combination chemotherapy increases toxicity to healthy cells as well as tumor cells.

The goal of combination chemotherapy is to select drugs that are *additive* in therapy and *subadditive* in toxicity.

II

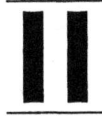

Routes of Administration

Chemotherapy is administered via a variety of routes. The specific route of administration depends upon a number of factors, including:

1. Type of chemotherapy (e.g., vesicant, biological properties)
2. Dosage of chemotherapy
3. Patient's health status (including venous status)
4. Patient's lifestyle
5. Resources available (technical and human)
6. Route and method drug is most effectively administered (e.g., does continuous infusion of drug cause fewer side effects than bolus? Is drug more effective if delivered directly to the target organ [e.g., liver] or given systematically [IV])?

The routes of administration include:

1. Oral
2. Subcutaneous
3. Intramuscular
4. Intravenous
5. Intra-arterial
6. Intrathecal
7. Intracavitary

Prior to the administration of any chemotherapeutic agent, a thorough patient assessment should be carried out. (Refer to Appendix III.)

Intravenous

The most common route of chemotherapy administration is the intravenous route. Delivery of drugs into the venous system through a peripheral line can include:

1. Bolus/direct push infusion
2. Through the side arm of free flowing IV
3. Piggyback into an established IV
4. By continuous infusion (recommended only if drug is a nonvesicant)

The following guidelines have been established by the Oncology Nursing Society for the peripheral administration of chemotherapy. They apply to all intravenous chemotherapy infusions.

1. Select the appropriate equipment.
2. Instruct the patient to remove obstructive clothing and jewelry or reposition identification band if necessary.
3. Examine the veins and solicit patient's opinions/wishes regarding site selection (see fig. 2.1A and 2.1B).
   - Proceed distally to proximally.
   - Avoid site of mastectomy, phlebitis, invading neoplasm, antecubital fossa, hematomas, lower extremities, varicosities, inflamed or sclerosed areas,

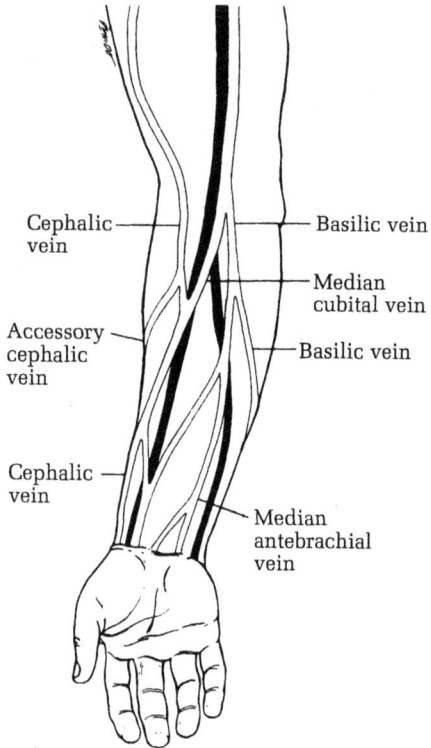

Cephalic vein

Basilic vein

Median cubital vein

Accessory cephalic vein

Basilic vein

Cephalic vein

Median antebrachial vein

Figure 2.1A.   Superficial veins of the forearm.

Memory Bank for Chemotherapy

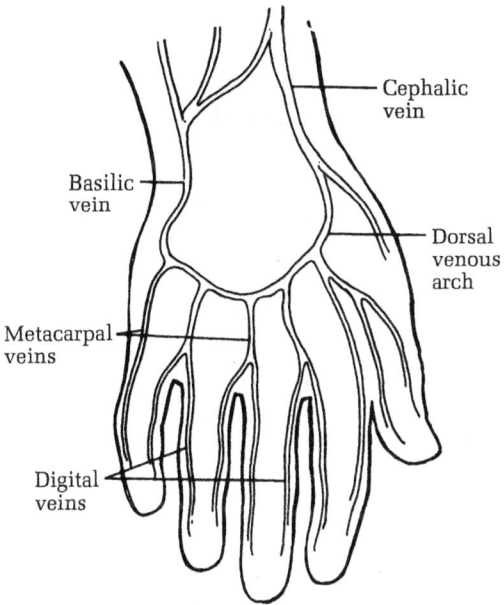

Figure 2.1B.   Superficial veins of the dorsal aspect of the hand.

impaired lymphatic drainage, impaired venous circulation, or sites distal to recent venipuncture.
- Alternate arms if possible.
- Avoid using existing peripheral intravenous lines.
- Use heat if necessary to distend veins.

4. Verify drug(s), doses, routes, and patient identification.
5. Wash hands.
6. Apply tourniquet.
7. Cleanse site according to the institutional policy and procedure.
8. Insert needle, observe blood backflow, remove tourniquet; tape needle to allow observation of insertion site.
9. Stabilize hand/arm; use arm board/pillow if necessary.
10. Infuse sterile normal saline/sterile distilled water.
11. Observe for infiltration continuously during bolus infusion; observe infusion site at least every 30 minutes for continuous infusions.
12. Administer drug(s) as ordered in accordance with the approved policy of the facility.
13. Observe site for swelling, redness, blebs, hives, etc.

14. Solicit patient's sensations (e.g., pain, burning, stinging) during treatment.
15. Reconfirm vein patency periodically (e.g., lower the IV bag and observe for blood return; aspirate until blood return is noted).
16. Provide sufficient amounts of sterile normal saline/sterile distilled water between drugs to completely flush the IV lines of residual drugs.
17. Observe patient continuously during and after treatment for adverse reactions.
18. Infuse sterile normal saline/sterile distilled water post-treatment.
19. Remove needle, apply sterile dressing.
20. Elevate the extremity and apply pressure for 3–5 minutes. Observe for hematoma after 5 minutes.
21. Apply Band-aid.
22. Dispose of equipment according to institutional policy.
23. Wash hands.
24. Document according to institutional policy and procedure.

Central (Vascular Access Devices)

Central lines are the best access devices for the continuous administration of chemotherapy, especially vesicant chemotherapy.

Right-Atrial Catheters

Right-atrial catheters (Hickman, Broviac, Corcath, Groshong) are pliable silicone catheters surgically inserted into a central vein (usually cephalic or external jugular) and advanced to the right atrium of the heart. They are tunnelled through subcutaneous tissue and exit at a site on the chest wall (see fig. 2.2). These catheters are used for intravenous infusions, medications, blood transfusion, nutritional support, and blood drawing. Care of these catheters varies among individual institutional policies but targets these main areas:

  a. Dressing change
  b. Catheter heparinization
  c. Catheter (injection) cap change

The following are examples of right atrial catheter care protocols:

Dressing Change

- Clean work area and wash hands.
- Assemble the following:
  - 3 alcohol swabsticks
  - 3 povidone-iodine swabsticks
  - 1 pre-slit sterile 2×2 gauze
  - 1 over dressing (e.g., bio-occlusive, 4×4 gauze)
  - 2 strips of 1-inch tape
  - povidone-iodine ointment (optional)

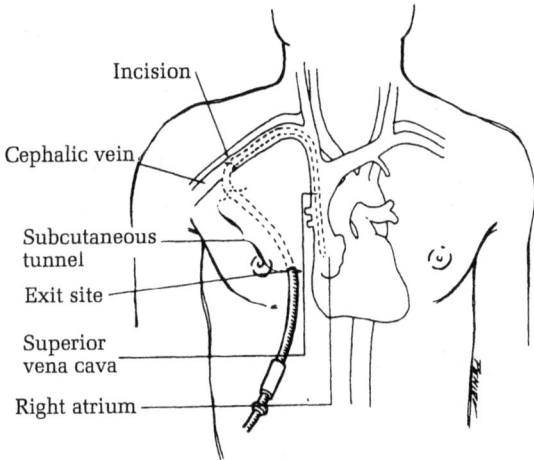

Figure 2.2. Right atrial catheter placement.

- Remove old dressing.
  - Remove tape and old dressing, taking care not to pull the catheter.
  - Inspect the exit site of the catheter for leakage, drainage, pus, swelling, redness.
  - Notify the patient's physician as soon as possible if any of the above signs are observed.

- Cleanse the skin.
  - Using alcohol swabs/swabsticks, cleanse the skin well from the exit site of the catheter, working outward in a circular motion. (Repeat two more times, using new swabstick each time.)
  - Use povidone-iodine swabsticks in the same manner as the alcohol swabstick.
  - Optional: Apply a small dab of povidone-iodine ointment to the exit site using a 2×2 gauze.
- Apply the new dressing.
  - Place the 2×2 gauze pad over the catheter having the catheter come through the slit.
  - Place dressing over the gauze pad and secure. Smooth the edges. (Tape the edges if they begin to curl.)
  - Coil catheter and tape to dressing.
- Frequency of dressing change is dependent upon institutional policy.

Catheter Heparinization
- Clean hands and work area.
- Open catheter clamp.
- Flush catheter with 10 cc NS followed by 3 cc heparin (100 units/cc).
- Reclamp catheter, coil, and tape in place.
- Flush after each use and monthly when not actively used. (Note: Multilumen catheters require more frequent flushings.)

Replacement of Catheter Injection Cap
- Clean hands and work area.
- Clamp catheter.
- Wipe the connection of the old catheter cap and catheter with a povidine-iodine wipe followed by an alcohol wipe.
- Carefully remove old cap.
- Reapply new cap and screw into place. (Do not touch the inside of the new cap.)
- Unclamp catheter, coil, and tape into place.

Nontunnelled Central Venous Catheters

Small gauge nontunnelled venous catheters are silicone elastomer catheters inserted either centrally (subclavian vein) or peripherally (brachial or cephalic) and advanced to the superior vena cava. They can be inserted at the patient's bedside. Their use is the same as the right atrial catheter, with some controversies over repeated use for blood drawing. Care of these catheters is generally the same as the right atrial catheters. Since the catheters are not tunnelled, they are more prone to infection and are not recommended for long-term use (see table 2.1).

Implantable Subcutaneous Ports

Implantable subcutaneous ports (Mediport, Infusaport, Port-a-cath, P.A.S. Port) are metal or plastic encased ports with rubber septums attached to a silicone catheter that is inserted

Table 2.1
Types of Venous Access Devices and Indications for Their Use

Silastic Atrial Catheters	Small-Gauge Central Venous Catheters	Implanted Ports
Frequent venous access required for blood sampling, blood products, therapy, etc.	Frequent venous access required for chemotherapy	Infrequent venous access required
TPN and antibiotic therapy	Infrequent blood sampling via peripheral vein	A young child: frequent venous access not required
Single-bolus injections of chemotherapy	Single-bolus injections of chemotherapy	Infrequent blood sampling required

Short- or long-term chemotherapy infusions (vesicant or nonvesicant)	Short-term infusion chemotherapy (2–3 months)	TPN, blood transfusions, fluid replacement, or antibiotics
Inpatient/outpatient chemotherapy infusion	Short-term infusion of vesicant chemotherapy	Short- or long-term chemotherapy
Significant other or patient capable of caring for device	Inpatient/outpatient infusion therapy	Inpatient/outpatient infusion of nonvesicant chemotherapeutic agents
Bone-marrow transplant recipient	Significant other or patient capable of caring for device	Patient physically unable to care for VAD[a]
Patient with leukemia	Brief life expectancy	Cosmesis/patient preference

Source: Goodman, M. et al. (1984). Venous access services. *Oncology Nursing Forum, 11*(5), 19. (Reprinted with permission.)
[a]VAD = venous access device

into a central vein (see table 2.2). These ports are surgically implanted under the skin (see fig. 2.3). Usage is the same as the right atrial catheter. Special Huber (noncoring) point needles are used to access these ports to prevent coring of the septum (see fig. 2.4). Care of these ports involves heparinization on a schedule individualized for the device (monthly versus weekly versus intermittently). Because the port is totally implanted, no dressing or cap change is required. Infection can occur if adequate cleansing of the skin site is not done prior to accessing.

Judicious flushing and heparinization of vascular access devices after each usage will reduce the risk of catheter clotting. This is especially important after blood drawing.

The following is an example of a protocol for use of implantable ports:

- Scrub the injection site.
  - Scrub injection site with three povidone-iodine swabsticks in a circular motion from center of septum to outer periphery.
  - Repeat using three alcohol swabsticks.
- Using sterile gloves, palpate the port site to locate the septum (in the exact center of the port). For conventional bolus therapy, a straight "noncoring" needle is recommended. For continuous or long-term

infusion, a right angle (90°) "noncoring" needle is recommended.

- Puncture skin and septum with needle held at 90° angle, perpendicular to the port. Needle entry and contact of the needle stop are discerned from the "feel" of the needle as it passes through the septum to the needle stop point.

    Caution: The needle must be held securely against the needle stop below the septum during these procedures to avoid injecting the drug into the subcutaneous tissue. Do not impart angular motion or twist the needle and syringe once in the septum. This action will cut the septum and create a drug leakage path.

- Many users will connect a micro extension set to the needle at this point. This has been particularly effective when long-term continuous infusion is the therapy given.

- Prior to injecting any drug, flush the port with 20 ml of normal saline, to check needle placement, as above.

- Inject the drug, applying consistent pressure.

- After each drug is injected, flush the ports with 20–30 cc normal saline solution.

- Heparinize the port with 3 cc (100 units/cc) of heparin solution after each treatment or per institutional protocol.

Table 2.2
Comparing Implantable Venous Access Systems

Trade Name	Infusaid[a]	MediPort[a]	Port-A-Cath
Reservoir			
Base diameter	4.76 cm	3.5 cm	2.54 cm
Height	1.58 cm	1.1 cm	1.35 cm
Catheter			
Length	50.8	50.0 cm	76.2
Lumen diameter	0.6 mm or 1.0 mm	0.5 mm, 1.0 mm, 1.5 mm	0.76 mm or 1.02 mm
Weight	12.1 gm	15 gm	28 gm
Volume	0.2 ml in port	0.5 ml in port with 0.5 mm catheter	0.4 ml in port

	0.0032 ml/cm in 0.6 mm catheter	1.0 ml in port with 1.0 mm catheter	0.4 ml in 0.76 mm catheter
	0.0081 ml/cm in 1.0 mm catheter	1.5 ml port with 1.5 mm catheter	0.6 ml in 1.02 mm catheter
Septum diameter	0.25" (7 mm)	0.5" (8 mm)	0.45" (11.4 mm)
Maximum number of punctures[b]	1,000	1,500–2,000	1,000–2,000
Company	Infusaid Corp., Norwood, MA	Cormed, Inc., Medina, NY	Pharmacia NuTech, Piscataway, NJ

Source: Wilkes, G. et al. (1985). Long-term venous access. American Journal of Nursing, 85, 796. (Reprinted with permission.)
[a]Double lumen available
[b]May vary, depending on size of needle used and technique in entering port

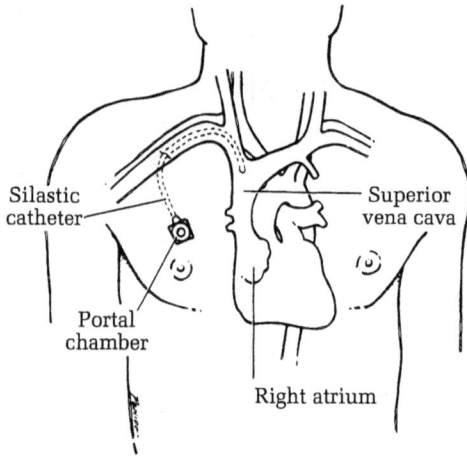

Figure 2.3.   Implantable ports.

Intra-arterial

The intra-arterial route of chemotherapy administration is done to provide direct infusion of a
chemotherapeutic agent to a specific site (e.g.,
intrahepatic arterial chemotherapy provides
direct perfusion of the liver) while sparing the
patient potentially toxic systemic side effects.
Intra-arterial chemotherapy can be delivered
intermittently or continuously via:

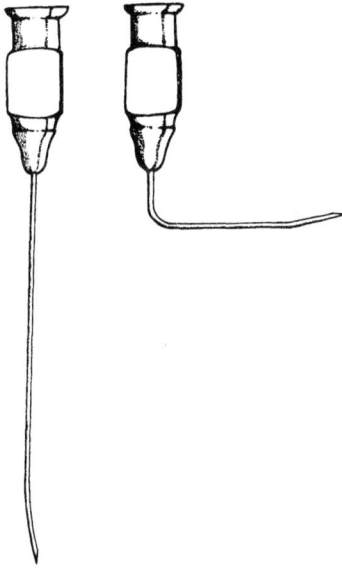

Figure 2.4. Huber point needles.

- Percutaneously placed arterial catheter (usually brachial)
- Surgically placed permanent arterial catheter attached to a small portable pump
- Surgically placed implantable pump (see figs. 2.5, 2.6)

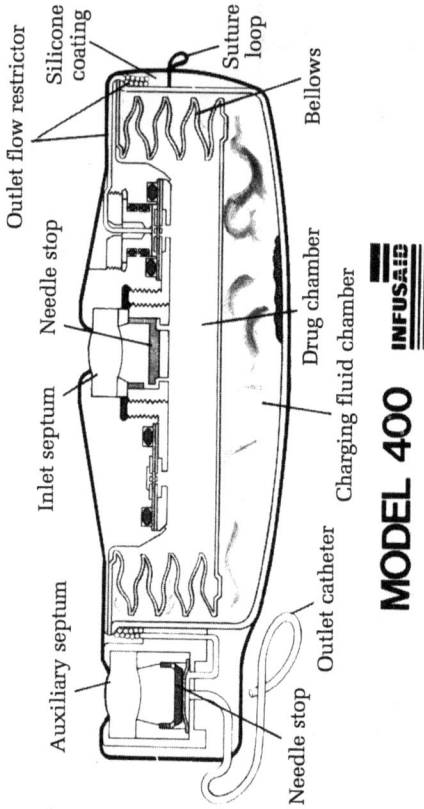

Figure 2.5. Infusaid pump (inner working).

Labels: Outlet flow restrictor, Silicone coating, Suture loop, Bellows, Needle stop, Drug chamber, Charging fluid chamber, Inlet septum, Auxiliary septum, Outlet catheter, Needle stop, MODEL 400, INFUSAID

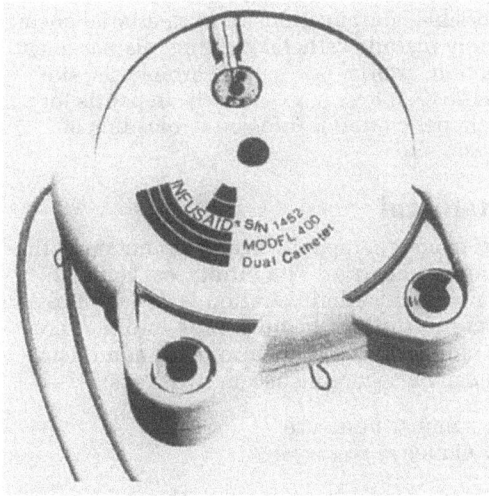

Figure 2.6. Infusaid pump.

Individual protocols determine the solution and fill time of the pump. When chemotherapy is not infusing, the pump is filled with heparinized saline. Patients must be taught to notify the health care team if they experience temperature changes or air pressure changes, as this will affect the pre-set drug delivery rate of the pump.

Possible complications of intra-arterial chemotherapy include catheter clotting, displacement, infection, arterial occlusion, thrombosis, site specific toxicities (e.g., gastritis, hepatitis for intrahepatic arterial infusions), bleeding at catheter site.

Intrathecal

Most chemotherapeutic agents do not cross the blood-brain barrier. The intrathecal route of chemotherapy administration is done to provide direct infusion of chemotherapy into the cerebral spinal fluid (CSF). Intrathecal administration can be accomplished in two ways:

1. Lumbar puncture
2. Ommaya reservoir

For repeated administration, the Ommaya reservoir is usually the preferred route, as it is less traumatic for both patient and certified nurse/MD administering the drug.

The Ommaya reservoir is a small plastic dome with an attached catheter. It is surgically placed under the scalp (usually in the right frontal region) and the catheter extends into a ventricle in the brain (see figs. 2.7, 2.8). The reservoir can be used for:

1. Administering medications into the cerebral spinal fluid
2. Withdrawing samples of cerebral spinal fluid for analysis
3. Measuring cerebral spinal fluid pressure

The reservoir is good for approximately 250 punctures.

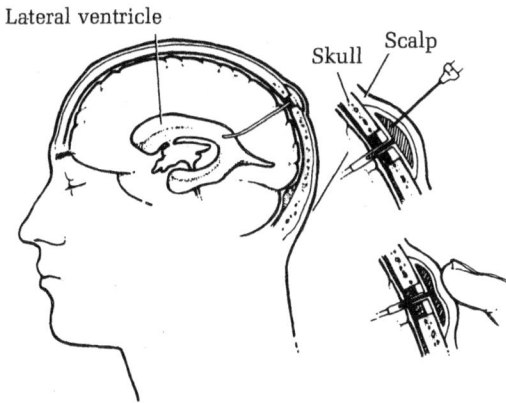

Figure 2.7.   CSF reservoir connected to lateral ventricle, showing mode of use.

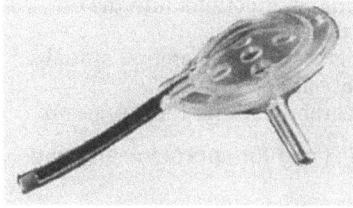

Figure 2.8. Ommaya reservoir.

Procedure for Administering Chemotherapy Via an Ommaya Reservoir

- Gently palpate site and assess for leakage.
- Prep site with three povidine-iodine swab-sticks using a circular motion.
- Prepare equipment.
- Don sterile gloves.
- Insert 23–25 gauge butterfly needle attached to an empty 5-cc syringe into the center of the Ommaya septum at a 45° angle.
  - Allow syringe to fill on its own. DO NOT ASPIRATE.
  - Remove syringe and send specimens as ordered.
  - Attach medication syringe and slowly administer (reconstitute medication with preservative-free NS).

- Remove medication syringe and attach syringe with preservative-free NS.
  - Flush reservoir.
- Remove needle and apply pressure to site for 2 minutes.

Possible side effects of intrathecal chemotherapy include headache, nausea and vomiting, dizziness, infection (meningitis), rapid onset of bowel movement, or diarrhea. These side effects, except meningitis, usually resolve on their own. Routine samples for occult infection should be sent to bacteriology. Prophylactic antiemetics should be administered when chemotherapy is given via an Ommaya reservoir.

Intracavitary

Intracavitary administration of chemotherapy involves the direct instillation of medication into an area of tumor involvement, thereby allowing a higher concentration of chemotherapy to be delivered to the site of disease. The three major sites treated in this manner are the thoracic cavity (pleural effusions), bladder, and peritoneum. The cavity is accessed via a catheter (e.g., Foley catheter, Tenckhoff, implantable port, thoracotomy tube, or angiocath). Chemotherapy is delivered through the catheter and allowed a dwell time. Dwell time is dependent upon the specific site and protocol and varies from 30 minutes to an indefinite period of time.

While only specially trained nurses should be administering intracavitary chemotherapy, it is the responsibility of all nurses caring for patients who have received intracavitary chemotherapy to monitor them for potential problems. These include:

1. Infection
2. Pain at site due to irritation (depends on agent used)
3. Change in respiratory status because of pressure on the diaphragm, if large quantities of fluid are instilled
4. Catheter complications (clotting, displacement)

III

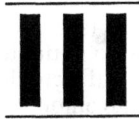

Administration of
Vesicants

Extravasation is the infiltration of intravenous fluids or drugs into the surrounding subcutaneous tissues. Vesicants (see table 3.1) are those drugs that have the potential to cause cellular damage when they infiltrate this subcutaneous tissue. Even a minute amount can cause damage, so special precautions must be taken when administering these vesicant agents. The vesicant drugs should only be administered by an MD or RN knowledgeable about the effects of chemotherapy.

Guidelines for Infusion of Vesicant Chemotherapy

1. A central line is preferable for administration of vesicants.
2. Start intravenous lines in the largest, straightest veins possible. Avoid extremities with impaired circulation or joints where sudden flexion is a possibility.
3. Caution patient regarding excessive movement while administration of drug is in progress.
4. Start a new IV site (with a butterfly or scalp vein) for administration, whenever possible.
5. Prior to drug administration, check patency and integrity of the IV.

Table 3.1
Vesicants

Dacarbazine (DTIC-Dome)

Daunomycin Hydrochloride
(Daunorubicin, Cerubidine)

Doxorubicin (Adriamycin-RDF)

Mechlorethamine (Mustargen)

Mitomycin (Mutamycin)

Plicamycin (Mithracin)

Vinblastine (Velban)

Vincristine (Oncovin)

     a. Lower the IV bag and note blood return
       from the IV.
     b. Note for the presence of redness,
       swelling, pain, or burning at site.
     c. Note positional change in the rate of the
       IV drip.
  6. Push vesicant drug slowly via the side arm
     of a rapidly running IV. Vigilant and clear
     observation of the IV site during
     administration is necessary.
     a. Check for local redness, swelling.
     b. Check with patient for symptoms of
       burning or pain.

Should extravasation occur, expedient, proper action is of the utmost importance. The treatment of extravasation of chemotherapy remains somewhat controversial. **It is recommended that each institution develop standing protocols so that treatment of suspected or actual extravasations can be instituted without delay.** The following protocols suggest treatments that could be followed.

Extravasation Protocols

Treatment of Extravasation of Nitrogen Mustard

1. Stop administration of the drug *immediately*.
2. Withdraw all remaining drugs in the IV tubing.
3. If the antidote (thiosulfate) or steroids are ordered, administer as ordered. To mix thiosulfate, add 6 cc of sterile water to a 10% sodium thiosulfate base (a 1/6 molar solution results). Usually, 5–6 cc of thiosulfate are injected through the existing IV tubing.
4. Discontinue IV.
5. Apply pressure and ice for 20 minutes every 4–6 hours × 72 hours.
6. Elevate extremity.
7. Notify MD.

8. Fill out an incident report or progress note in order to document what action was taken, appearance of the site, and any follow-up action to be taken.
9. Provide telephone follow-up within the first week to provide site assessment.
10. Administer analgesia as necessary.

Treatment of Extravasation of Vinca Alkaloids (Vincristine, Vinblastine, Vindesine)

1. Stop administration of the drug *immediately.*
2. Withdraw all remaining drugs in the IV tubing.
3. Discontinue the IV.
4. Administer hyaluronidase (Wydase) 1–6 cc (150–900 units) subcutaneously into extravasated site if ordered.
5. Apply pressure and warm soaks to the area for 20 minutes every 4–6 hours × 72 hours.
6. Elevate extremity.
7. Notify the MD.
8. Fill out an incident report or progress note to document what drug extravasated, what action was taken, what the site looked like, and any follow-up action to be taken.

9. Provide telephone follow-up within the first week to provide site assessment.
10. Administer analgesia as necessary.

Treatment of Extravasation of Other Vesicants (Non-vinca Alkaloids, Adriamycin, Mitomycin C, Plicamycin)

1. Stop administration of the drug immediately.
2. Withdraw all remaining drugs in the IV tubing.
3. Discontinue the IV.
4. Apply pressure and ice ASAP.
5. Elevate the extremity.
6. Notify the MD.
7. Administer a steroid (IV and/or topical) if ordered.
8. Fill out an incident report or progress note to document what drug extravasated, what action was taken, the appearance of the IV site, and follow-up action to be taken.
9. Provide telephone follow-up within the first week to provide site assessment.
10. Administer analgesia as necessary.

IV

Chemotherapeutic Agents

Boldface in Side Effects designates those most commonly occurring

Aldesleukin (Proleukin)

Class

Biological Response Modifier

Indications

Metastatic renal cell carcinoma, metastatic melanoma

Dosages

600,000 IU/kg every 8 hours for a total of 14 doses. Repeat in 10 days for a total of 28 doses.

Reconstitution

1.2 ml sterile water for injection for a concentration of 18 million IU/ml.
Do not shake vial.
Further dilute in 50 cc D_5W for infusion.

Administration

Infuse over 15 minutes

Stability

Check package for expiration date.
Store at room temperature. Use reconstituted vial within 48 hours.

Side Effects

Anemia, cardiac toxicities (capillary leak syndrome, hypotension, sinus tachycardia), pulmonary toxicities (dyspnea, edema), gastrointestinal toxicities (nausea, vomiting, diarrhea), fever, chills

Nurse Alert

- Patients with cardiac, pulmonary, CNS, hepatic, or renal impairment are at increased risk for serious and potentially fatal side effects/toxicities.

Aminoglutethimide (Cytadren)

Class

Miscellaneous
Cell Cycle Nonspecific

Indications

Cancer of the breast or prostate, adrenal
cortical carcinoma, ACTH-producing
ectopic tumors (drug provides a "medical
adrenalectomy")

Dosages

Vary according to individual protocols.
750 mg–2 gm PO every day in divided doses
250 mg PO every 6 hours

Reconstitution

None

Administration

Oral, available in 250 mg tablets

Stability

Check package for expiration date.

Side Effects

Anorexia, **dermatologic reaction (rash
with/without fever), fatigue,** gastrointestinal
alterations (nausea and vomiting), hepatic

toxicity (increased alkaline phosphatase, bilirubin, SGOT), **metabolic alterations (adrenal insufficiency,** hypothyroidism, decreased aldosterone level, decreased cortisol level), **neurotoxicity (ataxia,** headache, **nystagmus, somnolence)**

Nurse Alert
- Nausea and vomiting usually decrease after 2 weeks of treatment.
- Rash is noted in about 50% of patients and will usually resolve itself in 1 week; if no resolution, discontinue.
- Postural hypotension can occur as a result of lowered aldosterone levels.
- Always administer with a steroid (hydrocortisone 40–100 mg PO daily in 4 divided doses; Florinef 0.1 mg PO every other day).
- Monitor for symptoms of adrenal insufficiency (hyponatremia, facial flushing).
- Tell patient to avoid alcohol as it may potentiate somnolence.

Asparaginase/L-Asparaginase (Elspar)

Class

Enzyme
Cell Cycle Specific

Indications

Acute lymphoblastic leukemia, lymphoma

Dosages

Vary according to individual protocols.
200 IU/kg daily for 28 days
6,000 IU/m^2 3 times a week for 3 weeks
1,000 IU/kg twice weekly
1,000 IU/kg daily for 2–20 days
Test dose: 1–2 units, IV/IM/subcutaneously

Reconstitution

IV: Dilute the 10,000-unit vial with 5 cc sterile
water or normal saline; final concentration
2,000 units/cc.
IM: Dilute the 10,000-unit vial with 2 cc
sterile water or normal saline; final concentration 5,000 units/cc.

Administration

IV through the side arm of a running IV over
no less than 30 minutes
IM injections in a single dose, volume not
exceeding 2 cc

Stability

Check package for expiration date.
Store sterile powder in refrigeration.
Use diluted drug within 8 hours.

Side Effects

Allergic reactions (anaphylaxis), anemia, anorexia, arthralgias, neurotoxicities (depression, somnolence, fatigue, coma, confusion, agitation, hallucinations varying from mild to severe, headache), hypofibrinoginemia and **depression of other clotting factors,** dermatologic reactions, **flu-like syndrome** (chills, **fever), gastrointestinal alterations** (abdominal cramps, **nausea, vomiting,** pancreatitis) hyperthermia, leukopenia, metabolic alterations, hepatic toxicities (abnormal liver function tests, serum albumin, cholesterol, total lipids, fatty changes in the liver and malabsorption syndrome), respiratory distress, Parkinson-like syndrome, thrombocytopenia

(continued)

Asparaginase (continued)

Nurse Alert

- Because of the high incidence of allergic reactions, intradermal skin testing is recommended prior to initial administration. A physician should always be present when the drug is being administered, however, reactions can occur as long as 2–24 hours after administration.
- Monitor vital signs immediately prior to, 15 minutes into infusion, and immediately following drug administration.
- Have epinephrine, diphenhydramine (Benadryl) and hydrocortisone at bedside.
- The *E. Coli* strain is used most often. The Erwinia strain is used if patient is allergic to *E. Coli asparaginase*.
- May not be used in maintenance therapy as tolerance to the drug may develop.
- Administered after vincristine and prednisone to decrease toxic effects, if these drugs are ordered.
- Hepatotoxicity may enhance any toxic side effects.
- Pancreatitis is a possible contraindication to the use of this drug.

Bleomycin Sulfate (Blenoxane)

Class

Antineoplastic Antibiotic
Cell Cycle Specific

Indications

Squamous cell carcinoma of the head and
neck, skin, penis, cervix, and vulva;
lymphomas, Hodgkin's disease, reticulum
cell sarcoma, lymphosarcoma, testicular
carcinoma, embryonal cell, choriocarcinoma,
teratocarcinoma.

Dosages

Vary according to individual protocols.
0.25–0.50 units/kg (10–20 units/m^2) weekly or
biweekly (1 unit = 1 mg)
Test dose: 1–2 units IM or intradermally

Reconstitution

For IV solution dilute 15-unit vial with 1–5 cc
of sterile water, sodium chloride, or D$_5$W.
For IM or subcutaneous injections, use 1 cc
and 0.5 cc diluent respectively.

(continued)

Bleomycin Sulfate (continued)

Administration

Give IV injections over 10 minutes via the side arm of a running IV or soluset. Administer IM and subcutaneous injections slowly. Intracavitary infusions are given for malignant effusions. Continuous infusions of 4–12 hours are given via intravenous or intra-arterial infusions.

Stability

Check package for expiration date.

Store under refrigeration. After reconstitution, stable for 4 weeks under refrigeration if reconstituted with bacteriostatic diluent.

Side Effects

Alopecia, anorexia, anaphylaxis (hypotension, mental confusion, **fever, chills**, and wheezing), **dermatologic reactions (erthema, rash, stria, vesiculation, hyperpigmentation,** skin tenderness, **hyperkeratosis,** nail changes, **pruritus**), gastrointestinal alterations (nausea, vomiting), pain at tumor site, **pulmonary complications (pneumonitis,** pulmonary fibrosis, dyspnea, rales, decreased pulmonary function), phlebitis, **stomatitis,** isolated cases of Raynaud's syndrome are seen in patients with testicular carcinoma who receive concomitant vincristine.

Nurse Alert
- Because of the high incidence of anaphylactic reactions in patients with lymphoma, a test dose of 1–2 units should be given for the first 2 doses.
- Patients greater than 70 years of age or who have received greater than 400 total units or who are status post-mediastinal radiation therapy should have serial pretreatment chest X-rays and pulmonary function tests.
- Avoid administration of high tension O_2 after bleomycin because of the increased risk of pulmonary fibrosis.
- IM and SC injections may cause pain, alert patient.
- Fever and chills can occur up to 6 hours after administration.
- If a known febrile response occurs, prophylactic steroids/acetominophen may be warranted.
- Have epinephrine, diphenhydramine (Benadryl), and hydrocortisone at bedside.

Busulfan (Myleran)

Class

Alkylating Agent
Cell Cycle Nonspecific

Indications

Chronic myelogenous leukemia, polycythemia
vera, myeloid metaplasia

Dosages

Vary according to individual protocols.
Induction: 2–12 mg/day PO for 3–4 weeks
Maintenance: 1–3 mg/day PO until an accept-
able WBC is achieved (usually 10,000–
20,000 mm^3)

Reconstitution

None: 2-mg tablets

Administration

Oral

Stability

Check package for expiration date.

Side Effects

Addisonian-like asthenia, anemia, cardiotoxicity (endocardial fibrosis), cataracts,
dermatologic reaction (dermatitis, skin

pigmentation), gastrointestinal alterations (nausea, vomiting, diarrhea), **gynecomastia, leukopenia, pulmonary toxicities (cough, dyspnea, interstitial pulmonary fibrosis),** reproductive dysfunction (amenorrhea, testicular atrophy, impotence), **thrombocytopenia**

Nurse Alert

- Drug may be administered with allopurinol to prevent hyperuricemia if uric acid is elevated.
- Instruct patient to drink 10–12 glasses of water daily.
- WBC continues to fall for 2–3 weeks after drug is discontinued.
- "Busulfan lung" is a syndrome of cough, dyspnea, and low-grade fever due to interstitial pulmonary fibrosis seen rarely with chronic long-term usage.

Carboplatin (Paraplatin)

Class

Alkylating Agent
Cell Cycle Nonspecific

Indications

Ovarian cancer, lung cancer

Dosages

Vary according to individual protocols.
360 mg/m² IV every 4 weeks

Reconstitution

Dilute with sterile NS or sterile water for
injection for concentration of 10 mg/ml.
May further reconstitute in D_5W or NS.

Administration

IV as a 2-hour infusion or continuous 24-hour
infusion

Stability

Check package for expiration date.
Reconstituted solutions are stable at room
temperature for 24 hours.

Side Effects

Anemia, **gastrointestinal alterations (nausea,
vomiting,** diarrhea), hepatic toxicities, **metabolic alterations (hyponatremia, hypocalcemia, hypokalemia, hypomagnesemia),**

neurotoxicity (ototoxicity, **paresthesias,** peripheral neuropathies), renal toxicity, anaphylaxis (rare), leukopenia, thrombocytopenia, alopecia, reproductive dysfunction (mutagenic)

Nurse Alert

- Aluminum containing needles and IV sets should not be used.
- Use caution with patients receiving other nephrotoxic drugs as their renal effects may be potentiated by Carboplatin.
- Bone marrow depression is dose related. Anemia may be cumulative.
- Due to high emetic potential of drug, premedicate with antiemetic therapy and continue for 24–48 hours post-treatment as necessary. Emesis is decreased when drug administered is over 24-hour continuous infusion or daily pulse dosing for 5 days.
- The Calvert formula (Total dose (mg) = (target AUC) × (GRF = 25) is often utilized for more individualized dosing.
- Dose not have the same renal toxicity as Cisplatinum.
- Have epinephrine, diphenhydramine (Benadryl), and hydrocortisone at bedside.

Carmustine/BCNU (BiCNU)

Class

Nitrosourea
Cell Cycle Nonspecific

Indications

Brain tumors (glioblastoma, brainstem glioma,
medulloblastoma, astrocytoma, ependy-
moma, metastatic brain tumors), multiple
myeloma, lymphoma, Hodgkin's disease,
lung cancer, malignant melanoma, gastric
cancer, mycosis fungoides (investigational
topical use)

Dosages

Vary according to individual protocols.
200 mg/m^2 IV every 6–8 weeks
75–100 mg/m^2 IV every day for 2 days, every
6–8 weeks

Reconstitution

Add 3 cc of provided diluent (alcohol) to the
100 mg vial.
Further dilute with 27 cc sterile water for
injection.
Final concentration is 3.3 mg/cc. Further
dilute in D$_5$W or normal saline in amount
sufficient for infusion. Do not use vial in
multidose fashion as it contains no
preservative.

Administration

Given as infusion over 1–2 hours. Shorter
infusion times may increase pain and
burning at the incision site.

Stability

Check package for expiration date.

Use with 2 hours of reconstitution if drug is
not refrigerated. Under refrigeration, the
reconstituted solution is stable for 24–48
hours.

Do not store in plastic bags or use them for
long-term infusions.

Side Effects

Anemia, **facial fushing, gastrointestinal
alteration (nausea, vomiting),** gynecomastia,
hepatic toxicity (jaundice; elevated SGOT,
alkaline phosphatase, bilirubin), **leukopenia, neurotoxicity (dizziness,** ataxia),
**pulmonary toxicity (fibrosis, dyspnea,
cough, chest pain),** renal toxicity (elevated
BUN), **thrombocytopenia**

(continued)

Carmustine (continued)

Nurse Alert

- Bone-marrow suppression is delayed (up to 6 weeks).
- Drug crosses the blood-brain barrier, which is why it is utilized in treatment of brain tumors.
- Oil film at/on bottom of drug vial indicates decomposition of drug and vial should be discarded.
- Pain along venous route during infusion can be decreased by increasing diluent, decreasing infusion rate, or placing ice above injection site.
- Rapid infusion of drug may result in facial flushing, dizziness.
- Hyperpigmentation and burning can result if drug is spilled on skin.

Chlorambucil (Leukeran)

Class

Alkylating Agent
Cell Cycle Nonspecific

Indications

Chronic lymphocytic leukemia, Hodgkin's
disease, lymphoma, cancer of the breast,
ovary, testes, choriocarcinoma,
Waldenström's macroglobulinemia,
thrombocythemia

Dosages

Vary according to individual protocols.
0.1–0.2 mg/kg every day for 3–6 weeks, then
2–6 mg every day
4–8 mg/m^2 day for 2–3 weeks

Reconstitution

None: 2-mg tablets

Administration

Oral

Stability

See package for expiration date (has a shelf
life of only 1 year).

(continued)

Chlorambucil (continued)

Side Effects

Anemia, cystitis, dermatologic reaction, gastrointestinal alteration (nausea, vomiting, diarrhea), hepatotoxicity, **leukopenia,** neurotoxicity (seizures, peripheral neuropathies), pulmonary toxicities (fibrosis, alveolar dysplasia), renal toxicity **(hyperuricemia),** reproductive dysfunction (amenorrhea, oligospermia, azoospermia), secondary malignancies (acute myelogenous leukemia), stomatitis, **thrombocytopenia**

Nurse Alert

- Drug is a derivative of nitrogen mustard.
- Leukopenia can be delayed up to 3 weeks.
- If drug is administered within 4 weeks of radiation therapy or chemotherapy, a dose modification may be indicated because of bone-marrow depression.
- Toxicities may be increased if drug is administered concomitantly with barbiturates.
- Tell patient to drink 10–12 glasses of water daily.

Cisplatin/CIS-DDP/CIS-Platinum II (Platinol)

Class

Miscellaneous
Cell Cycle Nonspecific

Indications

Carcinomas of the testes, ovary, bladder, lung, head and neck, prostate, esophagus, and cervix, Hodgkin's disease, non-Hodgkin's lymphomas, melanoma, osteosarcomas

Dosages

Vary according to individual protocols.
50–120 mg/m^2 IV every 3–4 weeks
15–20 mg/m^2 IV daily × 5 days every 3–4 weeks
20–120 mg/m^2 for intra-arterial administration

Reconstitution

Dilute with sterile water for injection for a concentration of 1 mg/cc. Further dilution should be in 0.9% or 0.45% saline in amounts dependent on the length of infusion.

Administration

IV, intra-aterial, intraperitoneal. Avoid rapid IV infusion. Intra-arterial administration may be given with heparin depending on institution protocol.

(continued)

Cisplatin (continued)

Stability

Check package for expiration date.
Store unreconstituted powder at room
temperature, protected from light.
Reconstituted solutions are stable at room
temperature for 20 hours and should not be
refrigerated.

Side Effects

Anemia, anaphylaxis (rare), anorexia, cardiotoxicity (rare), hepatotoxicity, leukopenia,
**metabolic alterations (hypomagnesemia,
hypocalcemia, hypokalemia, hypophospha-
temia,** hyperuricemia), **gastrointestinal
alterations (nausea, vomiting), neurotoxicity
(ototoxicity,** paresthesias), reproductive dysfunction (mutagenic and teratogenic properties), **renal toxicities,** thrombocytopenia,
phlebitis

Nurse Alert

- Monitor renal status; check BUN, serum
  creatinine, uric acid levels, and creatinine
  clearance prior to administration.
- Give with vigorous pre- and posthydration
  with normal saline with or without diuretics
  (e.g., mannitol, furosemide).

- Maintain urinary output at 100 cc/hour during administration and posthydration periods.
- Monitor for fluid overload.
- Cisplatin has high emetogenic properties; premedicate with antiemetic therapy and continue for 48–96 hours post-therapy as necessary.
- Establish audiologic baseline studies prior to initial treatment to monitor ototoxicity.
- Do not administer through an aluminum needle (platinum reacts with aluminum).
- Anaphylactic-like reactions have been known to occur within a few minutes of administration.
- WBC and platelet nadir is approximately 2 weeks after treatment.
- Check electrolyte levels (calcium, potassium, phosphates, magnesium) prior to each administration; hypomagnesemia is particularly common.
- Aminoglycosides, amphotericin B, and methotrexate can potentiate cisplatin-related nephrotoxicity.
- Have epinephrine, diphenhydramine (Benadryl), and hydrocortisone at bedside.

Cyclophosphamide (Cytoxan, Neosar)

Class

Alkylating Agent
Cell Cycle Nonspecific

Indications

Malignant lymphoma, Hodgkin's disease,
multiple myeloma, leukemias, cancer of the
breast, prostate, lung, uterus, ovary, and
testes, mycosis fungoides,
rhabdomyosarcoma, neuroblastoma,
retinoblastoma

Dosages

Vary according to individual protocols.
50–100 mg/m^2 PO daily
500–1,500 mg/m^2 IV every 3–4 weeks

Reconstitution

Dilute with sterile water for injection to a
concentration of 5 cc for every 100 mg of
drug for a final concentration of 20 mg/cc.
Bacteriostatic water may be used if the
preservative is parabens; do not use benzyl-
alcohol preserved water.
Also available in 50-mg tablets.

Administration

IV, PO, intrapleural, or intraperitoneal

Stability

Check package for expiration date.

Stable at room temperature for 24 hours or refrigerated for 6 days if diluent contains a preservative.

Side Effects

Alopecia (increased with IV administration), anemia, anorexia, cardiac toxicity, hemorrhagic cystitis, hepatic toxicity, **leukopenia, gastrointestinal alterations (nausea, vomiting),** metabolic alterations (hyponatremia), renal toxicity, reproductive dysfunction (azoospermia, amenorrhea, sterility), secondary malignancies (bladder cancer, leukemia), sexual dysfunction (impotence, decreased libido), thrombocytopenia

Nurse Alert

- Tell patient to take the PO dose early in the day to assure adequate hydration and prevent bladder stasis.
- IV doses greater than 500 mg/m^2 IV push have a higher incidence of dizziness, rhinorrhea, flushing, and diaphoresis.
- Pre- and post-treatment hydration (100–300 cc) are recommended with IV doses.

(continued)

Cyclophosphamide (continued)

- May potentiate doxorubicin-induced cardiotoxicity.
- May interfere with normal wound healing.
- High IV doses may have antidiuretic effect; monitor sodium levels for hyponatremia.
- Allopurinol and thiazide-type diuretics potentiate side effects of cyclophosphamide.
- Cyclophosphamide must be metabolized by the liver before it is activated, therefore liver function tests must be monitored for potential dose modification.
- Chronic administration of barbiturates increases the metabolism and the leukopenic activity of cyclophosphamide.

Cytarabine/Cytosine Arabinoside/ARA-C (Cytosar-U)

Class

Antimetabolite
Cell Cycle Specific

Indications

Acute myelogenous and lymphocytic
leukemia, lymphoma, head and neck cancer

Dosages

Vary according to individual protocols.
Leukemia: Induction 100–200 mg/m^2 IV by
continuous infusion for 5–7 days
100 mg/m^2 IV, subcutaneously every 12 hours
for 7–21 days
High dose: 1.5–4.5 gm/m^2 IV every 12 hours
for 2–6 days
Head and neck cancer: 1 mg/kg IV,
subcutaneously every 12 hours for 5–7 days
Intrathecal: 20–30 mg/m^2 every 4 days until
CSF is normal. Total dose usually not to
exceed 30 mg

(continued)

Cytarabine (continued)

Reconstitution

Use diluent provided for the following concentrations:

Add 5 cc diluent to the 100-mg vial for final concentration of 20 mg/cc.

Add 10 cc diluent to the 500-mg vial for final concentration of 50 mg/cc.

Do not reconstitute with provided diluent if drug is to be administered in high doses or intrathecally as the diluent provided in the package contains benzyl alcohol and could produce neurologic effects; use preservative-free diluent.

Administration

IV, IM, intrathecally, or subcutaneously. IV doses are usually administered over 1 hour; high doses over 1–3 hours.

Stability

If reconstituted with diluent provided in packet, the drug is stable for 48 hours.

If reconstituted with preservative-free diluent (for high dose or intrathecal use), administer soon after diluting and discard unused portion.

Side Effects

Alopecia, **anemia, anorexia,** "cytarabine syndrome" (chest pain, fever, arthralgias, headache, malaise), dermatologic reaction **(anal ulceration/inflammation, maculopapular rash on hands and feet,** photosensitivity), **gastrointestinal alterations (nausea, vomiting, diarrhea),** hepatic toxicity, **leukopenia,** metabolic alterations (hyperuricemia), neurotoxicity (headache, meningitis, paraplegia, ataxia, dysarthria, necrotizing leukoencephalopathic syndrome, decreased motor coordination/strength), ocular reaction (photosensitivity, hemorrhagic conjuctivitis, decreased visual acuity, increased lacrimation, burning), **stomatitis, thrombocytopenia,** thrombophlebitis

Nurse Alert

- Neurotoxicities are usually seen with high doses and seem to increase with age and if the person is receiving concomitant central nervous system radiation therapy.
- "Cytarabine syndrome" appears 6–12 hours after infusion and responds to corticosteroids.

(continued)

Cytarabine (continued)

- All toxicities appear to be dose related with the greatest frequency occurring in patients receiving high dose.
- Toxicities may be increased with prolonged infusions.
- Dose modifications may be needed in patients with decreased liver function.
- Pancreatitis has been reported in patients who have had prior treatment with L-asparaginase.
- Subcutaneous injections may cause pain at the site.

Dacarbazine (DTIC-Dome)

Class

Alkylating Agent
Cell Cycle Nonspecific

Indications

Malignant melanoma, Hodgkin's disease, soft
tissue sarcomas, neuroblastomas, malignant
glucagonomas

Dosages

Vary according to individual protocols.
2–4.5 mg/kg daily × 10 days every 4 weeks
100–250 mg/m^2 daily × 5 days every 3 weeks
Hodgkin's disease: 150 mg/m^2 daily × 5 days
every 4 weeks or 375 mg/m^2 on day 1 every
15 days

Reconstitution

Dilute 100-mg vial with 9.9 cc of sterile water
and 200-mg vials with 19.9 cc of the same
diluent. Final concentration = 10 mg/cc.
Further dilution with appropriate amounts of
sodium chloride solution is necessary to
prevent irritation to the vessels.

Administration

Intra-arterial and IV administration only.
Administer over 20–30 min in adequate
diluent of 250–300 cc.

(continued)

Dacarbazine (continued)

Stability

Check package for expiration date.

Sterile powder is sensitive to light and heat and must be stored in the refrigerator. Reconstituted drug is stable in refrigerator for 72 hours and at room temperature for 8 hours.

If drug is diluted further, it is stable for 24 hours under refrigeration.

Side Effects

Anaphylaxis, anorexia, **alopecia,** dermatologic reactions (facial flushing, photosensitivitiy, urticaria erythema), **flu-like syndrome (malaise, headache, myalgias), gastrointestinal alterations** (diarrhea, **nausea, and vomiting), hepatic necrosis, leukopenia,** neurotoxicity (facial paresthesias), **thrombocytopenia**

Nurse Alert

- The drug is an irritant and needs to be thoroughly diluted (250–500 cc may be warranted) to ensure patient comfort, as severe burning at the site can occur.
- Infusion over 20–30 min is recommended rather than IV push.
- If infiltration occurs, apply warm compresses for 72 hours.
- Monitor liver function regularly.

Dactinomycin/Actinomycin D (Cosmegen)

Class

Antibiotic
Cell Cycle Nonspecific

Indications

Choriocarcinoma, Wilms' tumor, Kaposi's sarcoma, Ewing's sarcoma, rhabdomyosarcoma, melanoma, testicular carcinoma, neuroblastoma, retinoblastoma

Dosages

Vary according to individual protocols.
15–30 mcg/kg/wk
10–15 mcg/kg/day × 5 days every 2–4 weeks
400–600 mcg/m^2 day × 5 days every 6–8 weeks
35–50 mcg/kg for isolated regional perfusion

Reconstitution

Mix 1.1 cc of sterile water for injection to 0.5-mg (500-mcg) vial for a final concentration of 0.5 mg/cc or 500 mcg/cc.
Do not use a diluent with a preservative as a precipitate may form.

(continued)

Dactinomycin (continued)

Administration

Administer through the side arm of a rapidly running IV; never give a direct IV bolus.

Has been administered intra-arterially for isolated regional perfusion.

Stability

Use within 24 hours of reconstitution due to lack of preservative in solution.

Drug is light sensitive.

Side Effects

Alopecia, anemia, anorexia, cardiac toxicity, dermatologic reacations (**acne, hyperpigmentation of previously radiated sites,** cheilitis), fatigue, **gastrointestinal alterations (nausea, vomiting, diarrhea,** proctitis, gastritis), hepatotoxicity (increased SGOT, hepatomegaly), **leukopenia,** secondary malignancies, **stomatitis, thrombocytopenia**

Nurse Alert

- Drug is an irritant; administer slowly.
- Dose modifications may be warranted if drug is administered concomitantly with radiation therapy as they can potentiate the effects of one another.
- Dosage is usually calculated in micrograms.

- Do not administer if patient is recovering from herpes zoster, or varicella as this could result in an exacerbation of the zoster virus.
- Premedicate with antiemetics as nausea and vomiting can be severe, however, they usually subside with successive daily doses.
- Leukopenia may be delayed up to 3 weeks after drug administration.
- Do not give through an in-line filter as binding occurs.

Daunomycin Hydrochloride
(Daunorubicin, Cerubidine)

Class

Antibiotic
Cell Cycle Nonspecific

Indications

Acute lymphoblastic and myeloblastic
leukemia, disseminated neuroblastoma

Dosages

Vary according to individual protocols.
30–60 mg/m^2/daily IV × 3–5 days every 3–4
weeks
25–45 mg/m^2 daily × 3–6 days

Reconstitution

4 cc of sterile water for injection to 20-mg vial
for a concentration of 5 mg/cc.
Can be further diluted with 10–15 cc normal
saline or D$_5$W.

Administration

Administer slow IV push over 2–5 min into
the side arm of a rapidly running IV.
Infuse over 5–10 min as a piggyback infusion
into a rapidly running IV under direct
constant supervision for any sign of
extravasation.

Stability

Check package for expiration date.

Store at room temperature. Use reconstituted vials within 24 hours if left at room temperature.

Side Effects

Alopecia, anemia, **cardiac toxicities** (congestive heart failure, cardiomyopathic ECG changes), **dermatologic reactions (general skin rash), fever, gastrointestinal alterations (nausea, vomiting),** hepatic toxicities (transient elevations of serum bilirubin, SGOT, alkaline phosphatase), **leukopenia, stomatitis, thrombocytopenia,** thrombophlebitis

Nurse Alert

- Drug is a potent vesicant and peripheral administration must always be done in the constant attendance of an MD or an RN knowledgeable in chemotherapy. Never administer the drug if the IV site is compromised. (See chapter 3.)
- May turn urine red.
- Cardiac toxicities may increase with a history of prior chest radiation therapy or concomitant cytoxan.

(continued)

Daunomycin Hydrochloride (continued)

- Do not mix with any other drugs.
- The total cumulative adult dose should not exceed 550 mg/m² without careful evaluation of the patient's cardiac status.
- Reduce dose in patients with impaired renal or hepatic function.

Doxorubicin (Adriamycin-RDF)

Class

Antibiotic
Cell Cycle Nonspecific

Indications

Acute leukemias, lymphoma, Hodgkin's
disease, small cell carcinoma of the lung,
hepatoma, gastric cancer, neuroblastoma,
sarcomas, Wilms' tumor, cancer of the ovary,
breast, prostate, thyroid, bladder, testicles

Dosages

Vary according to individual protocols.
60–75 mg/m^2 IV every 3 weeks
40 mg/m^2 IV on days 1 and 8 every 3 weeks
60–90 mg/m^2 IV over 24–96 hours as
continuous infusion every 3–4 weeks
25 mg/m^2 a day for 3 days intra-arterial
0.2–0.3 mg/kg intra-arterial for 2–20 days as a
continuous infusion
50 mg in 150 normal saline to be instilled into
bladder and retained for 30 min every 4
weeks.

Reconstitution

Dilute with sterile water or normal saline for a
final concentration of 2 mg/cc.

(continued)

Doxorubicin (continued)

Administration

IV push into the side arm of a rapidly running IV.

Infuse over 5–10 min as piggyback infusion with constant observation for extravasation.

Never administer as a direct IV bolus.

Stability

Check package for expiration date.

Reconstituted drug is stable at room temperature for 24 hours and in refrigeration for 48 hours.

Side Effects

Alopecia, anemia, anorexia, **cardiotoxicities,** diarrhea, flu-like syndrom (rare), **gastrointestinal alterations (nausea, vomiting,** diarrhea), dermatologic reactions, **leukopenia, stomatitis, thrombocytopenia**

Nurse Alert

- Drug is a potent vesicant and peripheral administration must always be done in the constant attendance of an MD or an RN knowledgeable in chemotherapy. Never administer the drug if the IV site is compromised. (See chapter 3.)
- If drug is to be administered as a continuous infusion, it must be done through a central venous catheter.

- Doses may be modified if used with con-comittant radiation therapy or in the presence of compromised cardiac or hepatobiliary function.
- Urine may be red after administration.
- WBC nadir is 10–14 days after administration.
- Doxorubicin is incompatible with heparin, 5FU, and dexamethasone; avoid mixing with any other drug.
- Dilute drug well to lower incidence of chemical phlebitis and dermatologic reactions.
- Can potentiate "radiation recall" (skin reactions of previously radiated sites).
- Cardiac toxicity and nausea and vomiting may be increased when drug is administered in combination with cyclophosphamide.
- Facial flushing may occur if the drug is given too rapidly.
- The total cumulative adult dose should not exceed 550 mg/m^2 unless serial cardiac ejection fractions are monitored closely.

Estramustine Phosphate Sodium (Emcyt)

Class

Miscellaneous
Cell Cycle Nonspecific

Indications

Prostatic carcinoma

Dosages

Vary according to individual protocols.
14–25 mg/kg/day PO in 3–4 doses
Usual dosage: 10–16 mg/kg/day

Reconstitution

None: 140-mg capsules

Administration

Oral

Stability

Check package insert for expiration date.
Store in refrigerator.

Side Effects

Anemia, anorexia, cardiac toxicity (hypertension, **fluid retention,** chest pain, peripheral edema, congestive heart failure,

myocardial infarction, cardiovascular
accident, pulmonary embolus), **dermatologic reaction (rash, pruritus), gastrointestinal alterations (diarrhea,
nausea/vomiting,** flatulence, bleeding),
gynecomastia, hepatic toxicity, leukopenia,
thrombocytopenia

Nurse Alert

- Administer cautiously to patients
  - with metastic bone disease (drug may
    influence metabolism of calcium and
    phosphorus),
  - with renal insufficiency or hypercalcemia,
  - with impaired hepatic function,
  - with thrombophlebitis (due to increased
    risk of thrombus formation),
  - with a cardiac history (congestive heart
    failure has been documented).
- Delayed nausea and vomiting can occur up
  to 8 weeks after the initiation of treatment.
- Take drug 1 hour before or 2 hours after
  milk or milk products. (Milk may affect the
  absorption.) Drug may be taken with meals
  to decrease nausea and vomiting.

Etoposide/VP-16 (VePesid)

Class

Mitotic Inhibitor
Cell Cycle Specific

Indications

Lymphoma, Hodgkin's disease, acute
nonlymphocytic leukemia, small cell lung
carcinoma, hepatoma, rhabdomyosarcoma,
Kaposi's sarcoma, cancer of the testicles,
bladder, prostate, uterus

Dosages

Vary according to individual protocol.
50–100 mg/m^2 IV × 5 days every 3–4 weeks
125 mg/m^2 IV on day 1, 3, and 5 every 4
weeks
Oral dose: 2 times the IV dose rounded to
nearest 50 mg, given on same schedule

Reconstitution

Mix in normal saline or D_5W in an amount
large enough to yield a concentration of
0.2–0.4 mg/cc.
Also supplied in 50-mg capsules.

Administration

IV over 30–60 min. Infusions of less than 30
min have resulted in broncospasms and
hypotension.

Stability

Check package for expiration date.

Reconstituted solutions (0.2 or 0.4 mg/cc) are stable for 48–96 hours respectively at room temperature.

Store capsules in refrigerator.

Side Effects

Alopecia, anaphylaxis, **anemia,** anorexia, flu-like syndrome, **gastrointestinal alterations (nausea, vomiting),** headache, **hypotension, leukopenia,** neurotoxicity, **thrombocytopenia**

Nurse Alert

- Anaphylactic-type reactions have been reported; have epinephrine, diphenhydramine (Benadryl), and hydrocortisone at bedside.
- Monitor blood pressure during infusion, every 15 min.
- WBC nadir usually occurs within 7–14 days after treatment and can be severe.

Floxuridine (FUDR)

Class

Antimetabolite
Cell Cycle Specific

Indications

Cancer of the head and neck, brain, liver
(primary or metastatic), gallbladder,
pancrease, bile ducts; solid tumors and
leukemias in children

Dosages

Vary according to individual protocols.
0.1–0.6 mg/kg daily intra-arterially for 1–6
weeks or until toxicity occurs

Reconstitution

500-mg vial is diluted with 5 cc sterile water
for injection to a concentration of 100
mg/cc. Further dilution can be with D_5W or
normal saline.

Administration

Intra-arterial
IV use is investigational.

Stability

Check package for expiration date.
Administer reconstituted solution within 24
hours; store in refrigerator, protect from
light.

Side Effects

Anemia, anorexia, dermatologic reactions
(skin sloughing on soles of feet and palms of
hands), **gastrointestinal alterations
(abdominal cramps, inflammation of the GI
tract, diarrhea, nausea, vomiting,** duodenal
ulcer, hiccoughs), **hepatic toxicity
(increased alkaline phosphatase, increased
bilirubin,** increased aminotransferase,
increased lactic dehydrogenase, sclerosis of
intra- and extra-hepatic bile ducts, chemical
hepatitis, abnormal prothrombin time,
sedimentation rate and total proteins),
leukopenia, metabolic alteration
(hypoadrenalism), neurotoxicity (lethargy,
nystagmus, vertigo, ataxia, blurred vision,
convulsions, mental depression,
hemiplegia), pain (localized to site of
infusion), **stomatitis,** thrombocytopenia

Nurse Alert

- Discontinue drug if intractable vomiting and
  diarrhea occur or at the first sign of
  mucositis.
- Use with extreme caution in patients with
  history of high-dose pelvic irradiation,
  treatment with alkylating agents, or with
  impaired liver or renal function.

(continued)

Floxuridine (continued)

- Drug is contraindicated in patients with poor nutritional status.
- Excreted via lungs and urine.
- Reported complications of intra-arterial infusion of chemotherapy have included
  - arterial problems (aneurysms, thrombosis, embolism, fibromyositis),
  - catheter site problems (blockage, displacement, leakage).

Fludarabine Phosphate (Fludura)

Class

Antimetabolite
Cell Cycle Specific

Indications

B-cell chronic lymphocytic leukemia (CLL),
non-Hodgkin's lymphoma

Dosages

Vary according to individual protocols.
25 mg/m^2 for 5 days every 28 days

Reconstitution

Add 2 ml sterile water for injection for concentration of 25 mg/ml.
Further dilute in 100 ml D_5W or NS for infusion.

Administration

IV over 30 min

Stability

Once reconstituted the drug should be used within 8 hours.

(continued)

Fludarabine Phosphate (continued)

Side Effects

Anemia, leukopenia, thrombocytopenia, gastrointestinal alterations (nausea, vomiting, anorexia, diarrhea, stomatitis), **malaise,** metabolic alterations (tumor lysis syndrome), peripheral edema, skin rash, neurotoxicity (weakness, parethesias, mental status changes), pulmonary (dyspnea, cough, infiltrates)

Nurse Alert

- Closely monitor patients for hemolysis. Reports of fatal autoimmune hemolytic anemia have been noted.
- Caution with dosages. High doses of Fludura have been associated with irreversible CNS toxicity including coma, blindness, and death.

Fluorouracil (Efudex, Fluoroplex)

Class

Antimetabolite
Cell Cycle Specific

Indications

Superficial basal cell carcinoma, malignant
lesions of the skin

Dosages

Apply cream over lesions 2 times daily for
3–12 weeks until lesions clear.

Reconstitution

None: 5% cream, IV solution to be applied
topically

Administration

Topical use

Stability

Check package for expiration date.

Side Effects

Dermatologic reactions (**burning,** hyperpigmentation, pruritus, **swelling of area
treated**), leukopenia, **pain in area treated,**
thrombocytopenia

(continued)

Fluorouracil (continued)

Nurse Alert

- Wear gloves when applying cream. Wash hands well after application.
- Avoid contact with eyes, nose, or mouth.
- Avoid occlusive dressing as it can increase the inflammatory response.
- Instruct patient to protect affected area from the sun with protective clothing and sun block.

Fluorouracil/5FU (Adrucil)

Class

Antimetabolite
Cell Cycle Specific

Indications

Cancer of the bladder, ovary, colon, rectum,
uterus, breast, cervix, pancreas, liver,
prostate, stomach, head and neck, pelvis;
malignant effusions, carcinoid

Dosages

Vary according to individual protocols.
500 mg–1.2 gm/m^2 IV daily × 5 days every
month
15 mg/kg IV weekly as maintenance
5 mg/kg/day intra-arterially for 4 days or until
toxicities develop
0.5 gm–3.0 gm intracavitary for pleural
effusions, peritoneal ascites, tumor seeding

Reconstitution

None; drug may be diluted in D$_5$W or normal
saline. If given intra-arterially it may be
mixed with heparin, depending on
institutional policy.

(continued)

Fluorouracil/5FU (continued)

Administration

IV, intra-arterial, intra-peritoneal, topical (see Efudex on page 89), oral (questionable efficacy). Drug can be given as a bolus or long- or short-term infusion.

Stability

Check package for expiration date.

Stable at room temperature.

Slight discoloration may occur but this does not affect drug potency. Exposure to low temperatures may cause precipitation in ampules. This can be dissolved by warming the ampule, shaking vigorously, or cooling to body temperature prior to use. Protect from long exposure to fluorescent light.

Side Effects

Alopecia, anemia, **anorexia,** cardiotoxicity (rare), dermatologic reactions (hyperpigmentation of nail beds and venous route, maculopapular rash on extremities, skin changes), **gastrointestinal alterations (diarrhea, nausea, vomiting),** increased lacrimation, **leukopenia,** neurotoxicity (photophobia, cerebral ataxia, **stomatitis, thrombocytoenia)**

Nurse Alert

- Monitor all stomata for signs of stomatitis (swelling, redness, pain, ulceration).
- Stomatitis or diarrhea may be the first signs of impending severe toxicities and should be an indicator to discontinue the drug.
- Fluorouracil is not compatible with doxorubicin, methotrexate, cytosine arabinoside, or diazepam (Valium).
- Patients who have had adrenalectomies may have increased requirements of cortisone therapy.
- WBC nadirs usually occur 9–14 days after treatment.
- Recommend sun block to avoid erythematous dermatitis.
- Caution patients receiving concomitant abdominal radiation therapy of the potential increase in gastrointestinal toxicities.

Flutamide (Eulixin)

Class

Antiandrogen

Indications

Prostate cancer

Dosages

Vary according to individual protocols.
250 mg every 8 hours

Reconstitution

None: 125-mg capsules

Administration

Oral

Stability

Check package for expiration date.
Store at room temperature.

Side Effects

Gastrointestinal (nausea, vomiting, diarrhea),
endocrine alterations (gynecomastia, galac-
torrhea), neurotoxicities (drowsiness, confusion, depression), hepatic toxicity (hepatitis),
sexual dysfunction (impotence, decreased
libido)

Nurse Alert

- Drug is given in conjunction with an LRHR
  agonist such as leuprolide.
- Inform patient hot flashes may occur.

Hexamethylmelamine
(HMM, ALTRETAMINE)

Class

Alkylating Agent
Cell Cycle Specific

Indications

Ovarian cancer

Dosages

Vary according to individual protocols.
4–12 mg/kg/day (divided into 3–4 doses) ×
21–90 days
6–8 mg/kg/day × 21 days every 6 weeks

Reconstitution

None: available in 50- to 100-mg capsules

Adminstration

Oral

Side Effects

Anemia, anorexia, **CNS toxicities** (confusion,
agitation, hallucinations), gastrointestinal
alterations (**nausea, vomiting,** diarrhea),
leukopenia, peripheral neuropathies,
pruritus, skin rash, thrombocytopenia

(continued)

Hexamethylmelamine (continued)

Nurse Alert

- Advise to take immediately after meals or in the middle of the meal to decrease nausea and vomiting.
- Concurrent B6 (pyridoxine) administration may decrease neurotoxicities.
- Nadir is 3–4 weeks post-treatment.
- May exacerbate neurotoxicities of other chemotherapies such as the vinca alkaloids.
- MAO inhibitors when given concomitantly can cause severe orthostatic hypotension.

Hydroxyurea (Hydrea)

Class

Miscellaneous
Cell Cycle Specific

Indications

Melanomas, chronic myelocytic and acute
leukemia; head and neck, ovarian, colon,
renal cell, prostate, lung, and gastric
carcinomas, polycythemia vera

Dosages

Vary according to individual protocols.
250 mg–3 gm/m^2 every 3 days
60–750 mg/m^2 daily
80 mg/kg every 3 days
20–30 mg/kg daily

Reconstitution

None: 500-mg capsules

Administration

Oral

Stability

Check package for expiration date.

(continued)

Hydroxyurea (continued)

Side Effects

Anorexia, anemia, alopecia, dermatologic reactions (**maculopapular rash,** facial erythema, pruritus, exacerbation of post-irradiation erythema), **leukopenia, gastro-intestinal alterations (nausea, vomiting, diarrhea,** constipation), neurotoxicities (headache, drowsiness, dizziness, disorientation, hallucinations, convulsions), renal toxicity (dysuria, hyperuricemia, uric acid stone development), **stomatitis, thrombocytopenia**

Nurse Alert

- High blood concentrations are achieved if the drug is given in 1 large daily dose rather than divided doses.
- If patient is unable to swallow, empty capsules into a glass of water and administer immediately; some inert particles may float undissolved on the surface.
- Administer with extreme caution to patients with impaired renal function (may rapidly develop auditory and visual hallucinations and severe hematologic toxicities).

Idarubicin (Idamycin)

Class

Antibiotic
Cell Cycle Specific

Indications

Acute myelogenous leukemia

Dosages

Vary according to individual protocols.
8–12 mg/m^2 daily for 3 days

Reconstitution

Add 5 cc NS to 5-mg vial
Add 10 cc NS to 10-mg vial
Yield: 1 mg/cc

Administration

Give IV push over 10–15 min into side arm of
rapidly running IV with constant observation for extravasation.

Stability

Check package for expiration date.
Reconstituted drug is stable at room temperature for 3 days and in refrigeration for 7
days.

(continued)

Idarubicin (continued)

Side Effects

Alopecia, anemia, gastrointestinal alterations (nausea, vomiting, anorexia, stomatitis), leukopenia, thrombocytopenia, cardiotoxicites, hepatic dysfunction, urticaria, hyperuricemia

Nurse Alert

- Drug is a potent vesicant. Peripheral administration must always be done in the constant attendance of an MD or RN knowledgeable in chemotherapy. Never administer the drug if the IV site is compromised. (See chapter 3.)
- If drug is to be administered as a continuous influsion it must be done through a central line.
- Urine may be red after administration.
- Use caution in patients with hepatic and/or renal dysfunction.
- Precipitation occurs when mixed with heparin.
- Cardiac toxicities are less common and severe than with doxorubicin and daunorubicin.

Ifosfamide (Ifex)

Class

Alkylating Agent
Cell Cycle Nonspecific

Indications

Germ cell cancer of the testicles, tumors
previously resistant to Cyclophosphamide

Dosages

Vary according to individual protocols.
1.5–2 mg/m^2 per day × 5 days every 3 weeks
1,200 mg/m^2 continuous infusion × 5 days
5,000 mg/m^2 IV single dose

Reconstitution

Dilute with SW or bacteriostatic water for
injection to a concentration of 1 gm/20 cc
for a final concentration of 50 mg/cc.

Adminstration

IV bolus over 30 minutes
IV infusion over 5 days

Stability

Check package for expiration date. Stable at
room temperature for 3 weeks if reconstituted with bacteriostatic water. Dilutions
prepared with preservative-free SW should
be used within 6 hours.

(continued)

Ifosfamide (continued)

Side Effects

Alopecia, CNS toxicity (somnolence, confusion), fever, gastrointestinal alteration **(nausea and vomiting), renal impairments** (hematuria), hepatic toxicity, leukopenia, phlebitis

Nurse Alert

- Use in combination with a prophylactic agent such as MESNA to prevent hemorrhagic cystitis.
- Monitor for hematuria.
- Force fluids to 2 L/day (po/IV).
- May interfere with wound healing.

Interferon Alfa-2b (Intron A)

Class
Biological Response Modifier
Immune Modulation
Direct Cytotoxic Effects; May Slow Cell Cycle

Indications
Non-Hodgkin's lymphoma, myeloma,
  melanoma, hairy cell leukemia, renal cell
  carcinoma, Kaposi's sarcoma, chronic
  myelogenous leukemia, carcinoid tumor,
  bladder cancer, ovarian cancer

Dosages
Low: 3×10^6 units/day
Moderate: 10×10^6 units/day
High: 30×10^6 units/day/m^2/3 times a week $\times$
  6 months

Reconstitution
Dilute with provided diluent or bacteriostatic
  water.

Administration
IM, IV, subcutaneous, intralesional

Stability
Stable for 1 month when reconstituted and
  refrigerated.
Check package for expiration date.
Store in refrigerator.

(continued)

Interferon Alfa-2b (continued)

Side Effects

Alopecia, anemia, changes in taste perception, **anorexia,** cardiotoxicity (ischemia, tachycardia, hypotension, dysrhythmias), dermatologic reaction (pruritus, dermatitis, dry skin, maculopapular rash), **flu-like syndrome (fever, chills, fatigue, myalgia, headache),** gastrointestinal alterations **(nausea/vomiting,** diarrhea, or constipation), hepatic toxicity (increased SGOT, SGPT), **leukopenia,** neurotoxicity (confusion, depression, somnolence paresthesias), thrombocytopenia

Nurse Alert

- Flu-like symptoms seem to decrease with continued administration.
- May exacerbate herpes lesions.
- Suggestion of a dose-response relationship (i.e., the higher the dose, the greater the tumor response).
- Administer at night so patient can sleep through side effects.
- Premedicate with acetaminophen and continue every 4 hours until no longer experiencing fever.

Leucovorin Calcium (Wellcovorin)

Class

Not a Cytotoxic Agent
Nutritional Supplement

Indications

A "rescue" after high dose or intrathecal
methotrexate.
Inhibits toxic effects of methotrexate that
would otherwise be lethal.
Use with 5FU as a potentiating agent.

Dosages

Vary according to individual protocols.
The dose is calculated depending on the dose
and route of methotrexate, creatinine clearance, and the serum methotrexate level.
Doses as high as 100 mg/m^2 every 3 hours
have been used; leucovorin "rescue" usually
begins 24 hours after the infusion of
methotrexate.

Reconstitution

Add 5 cc sterile water to 50-mg vial for a
concentration of 10 mg/cc. For IM use add
2.5 cc sterile water to 50-mg vial for a
concentration of 20 mg/cc. *Oral:* 5- and
25-mg tablets.

(continued)

Leucovorin Calcium (continued)

Administration

Oral, IM, IV

Stability

Check package for expiration date.
Reconstituted soution is stable for 7 days at
room temperature.

Side Effects

Allergic sensitization

Nurse Alert

- The importance of taking the correct dose at
  the correct times for an entire course cannot
  be emphasized too strongly.
- Thorough assessment of patient's ability to
  take oral leukovorin must be made as
  missing a dose could result in potentially
  lethal toxicities; patient may need to utilize
  parenteral route.
- Give with increased fluids and urine
  alkalization (e.g., sodium bicarbonate) to
  decrease potential nephrotoxicity.
- Patients discharged on oral leucovorin must
  have instructions regarding parenteral
  routes if they are unable to retain the
  tablets.

Leuprolide Acetate (Lupron)

Class

Antihormone

Indications

Prostate cancer

Dosages

Vary according to individual protocols.
1 mg SC daily
Lupron Depot: 7.5 mg IM every 28 days.

Reconstitution

No reconstitution necessary for SC Lupron.
Add 1 cc provided diluent to 7.5-mg vial of
   Lupron Depot for yield of 7.5 mg/cc.

Administration

SC, IM

Stability

Store syringes in refrigerator. Do not freeze.
Reconstituted Lupron Depot may be stored at
   room temperature for 24 hours.

Side Effects

Hot flashes, gynecomastia, gastrointestinal
   alterations (nausea, vomiting, diarrhea),
   neurotoxicities (dizziness, insomnia, par-
   esthesia), peripheral edema, sexual
   dysfunction (decreased libido, erectile
   impotence)

(continued)

Leuprolide Acetate (continued)

Nurse Alert

- Patients need to be instructed in proper administration techniques of Lupron.
- Initially patients may notice tumor flare and bone pain due to transient increase in LH secretion. This usually subsides in 2–3 weeks.
- Only reconstitute Lupron Depot with the diluent provided.

Lomustine/CCNU (CEENU)

Class

Nitrosourea
Cell Cycle Nonspecific

Indications

Tumors of the central nervous system;
   Hodgkin's disease and non-Hodgkin's
   lymphoma; melanoma; breast, renal,
   gastrointestinal, and lung carcinomas; used
   topically in the treatment of psoriasis and
   mycosis fungoides

Dosages

Vary according to individual protocols
130 mg/m^2 as a single dose every 6 weeks
100 mg/m^2 as a single dose every 6 weeks if
   patient's bone-marrow is suppressed

Reconstitution

None: 10-, 40-, 100-mg capsules

Administration

Oral

Stability

Check package for expiration date.
Store at room temperature.

(continued)

Lomustine (continued)

Side Effects

Alopecia, anorexia, anemia, **gastrointestinal alterations (nausea, vomiting),** hepatotoxicities, **leukopenia,** neurotoxicities (disorientation, lethargy, ataxia, dysarthria), pulmonary toxicities (infiltrates or fibrosis), renal toxicities, **stomatitis, thrombocytopenia**

Nurse Alert

- Monitor liver function tests periodically.
- Myelosuppressive effects occur late and dose intervals should be at least 6 weeks apart.
- Give drug on an empty stomach.
- Emesis can occur 45 min to 6 hours after administration. Drug may be given at bed time so patient can sleep through this discomfort.
- Vomiting usually occurs after the drug is absorbed, so there is no need to repeat the dose unless vomiting occurs immediately after ingestion of the drug.
- Premedication with antiemetics may be warranted.

Mechlorethamine/Nitrogen Mustard/HN$_2$ (Mustargen)

Class

Alkylating Agent
Cell Cycle Nonspecific

Indications

Hodgkin's disease and non-Hodgkin's lymphoma; mycosis fungoides; malignant effusions; bronchiogenic carcinomas such as epidermoid and small cell carcinomas; palliative treatment in carcinomas of the breast and ovary; chronic lymphocytic leukemia and polycythemia vera; emergency treatment of thrombocythemia

Dosages

Vary according to individual protocols.
0.4 mg/kg as a single dose or 0.1–0.2 mg/kg daily in divided doses every 3–6 weeks.
MOPP regimen: 6 mg/m^2, days 1 and 8 of a 28-day cycle
Intracavitary: 0.4 mg/kg
Intrapericardially: 0.2 mg/kg (10–20 mg)
Topical application: 10 mg dissolved in 60 cc of sterile water and applied daily, or once or twice a week per specific protocol

Reconstitution

Add 10 cc of sterile water or normal saline to each 10-mg vial for a l mg/cc concentration.

(continued)

Mechlorethamine (continued)

Administration

Wear protective gloves during administration of this drug because of the extreme irritation it causes to tissues. It should be pushed slowly (2–5 min) via the side arm of a rapidly running IV. Flush thoroughly for 2–5 min after administration.

Intracavitary infusion: Administer via a thoracentesis or paracentesis needle or catheter slowly, with frequent aspiration to ensure free flow of fluid.

Stability

Check package for expiration date. Store vials at room temperature. Use reconstituted solution within 15 min or discard due to rapid decomposition of drug.

Side Effects

Alopecia, **anemia,** anorexia, **burning sensation along vein,** dermatologic reaction (maculo-papular skin eruptions, erythema multi-forma), **fever, gastrointestinal alterations** (diarrhea, **nausea, vomiting,** peptic ulcer), **leukopenia,** neurotoxicities (weakness, headache, drowsiness, vertigo, convulsions, progressive muscle paralysis, paresthesias, cerebral degeneration, coma), hepatic toxicity (jaundice), ototoxicity (tinnitus, diminished hearing), reproductive toxicity (menstrual irregularities, impaired spermatogenesis), renal toxicity (hyperuricemia, hematuria), **thrombocytopenia**

Nurse Alert
- Wear double protective gloves during mixing. Never give drug IM or subcutaneously as severe necrosis will occur.
- Drug is a potent vesicant and peripheral administration must always be done in the constant attendance of an MD or an RN knowledgeable in chemotherapy. Never administer the drug if the IV site is compromised. (See chapter 3.)
- Because of its high emetogenic properties, adequate premedication with antiemetics and sedatives is necessary.
- Inhalationof dust or vapors and contact with the powder or solution of the drug with skin and mucous membranes must be avoided.
- Equipment (e.g., needles, gloves, vials, IV solutions) and unused solution must be neutralized with equal volume of 5% sodium thiosulfate and 5% sodium bicarbonate in water and allowed to soak for 45 min prior to disposal.

Medroxyprogesterone
(Depo-Provera, Provera)

Class

Hormone
Progestin

Indications

Renal cell, breast, endometrial, prostate cancer

Dosages

Vary according to individual protocols.
400–800 mg IM every week or month
Provera (the oral equivalent): 20–80 mg PO
every day

Reconstitution

None: 2.5-, 5-, 10-mg tablets
Ready to use solution: 100 or 400 mg/cc

Administration

IM, oral

Stability

Check package insert for expiration date.

Side Effects

Alopecia, **fluid retention,** gastrointestinal alterations (nausea and vomiting), **gluteal abscess (with IM injections), hepatoxicity (increased LFT),** hypersensitivity (local and usually due to reaction towards oil carriers of IM preparation), **metabolic alteration (increased calcium), weight gain**

Nurse Alert

• Use cautiously in patients with liver disease as drug is metabolized by the liver.

Megestrol Acetate (Megace, Pallace)

Class

Hormone
Progestin
Appetite Stimulant

Indications

Breast, endometrial, prostate, and renal cell
cancer

Dosages

Vary with individual protocols.
40–80 mg PO 1–4 ×/day (maximum of 320
mg/day)
800 mg/day for appetite

Reconstitution

None: 20- to 40-mg tablets
20 mg/cc liquid

Administration

Oral

Stability

Check package for expiration date.
May be stored at room temperature.

Side Effects

Alopecia, **breast tenderness,** dermatologic reaction (generalized rash), gastrointestinal alterations (nausea, vomiting, stomach cramps), hepatic toxicity (jaundice), neurotoxicity (headache), **reproductive dysfunction (vaginal bleeding, amenorrhea),** venous phlebitis, weight gain

Nurse Alert

• Same as medroxyprogesterone

Melphalan/L-Phenylalinine Mustard/L-Pam/L-Sarcolysin (Alkeran)

Class

Alkylating Agent
Cell Cycle Nonspecific

Indications

Multiple myeloma; ovarian, breast, prostate, testicular cancer; melanoma; chronic myelogenous leukemia; osteogenic sarcoma

Dosages

Vary according to individual protocols.
$10/mg/m^2$ PO for 4–7 days every 4–6 weeks
1 mg/kg PO every 4–6 weeks
6 mg PO every day until blood count stabilizes, then 2 mg PO every day for maintenance

Reconstitution

2-mg tablets

Administration

Oral

Stability

Check package for expiration date.
Store at room temperature.
Reconstituted IV solution is stable for 24 hours.

Side Effects

Alopecia, **anemia,** dermatologic reactions (rash, pruritus), gastrointestinal alterations (diarrhea, nausea and vomiting), **leukopenia,** pulmonary toxicity (bronchopulmonary dysplasia, interstitial fibrosis), reproductive dysfunction (amenorrhea, oligospermia), **secondary malignancies (leukemia),** stomatitis, **thrombocytopenia**

Nurse Alert

- Dose adjustments may have to be made in patients with impaired renal function.
- Blood count nadir may be prolonged up to 6 weeks in some patients with what seems to be a false recovery at about day 25.
- Drug is best taken on an empty stomach for better absorption.
- When a drug is administered parenterally (IV or intra-arterially) it should be treated as a vesicant.

Mercaptopurine/6-MP (Purinethol)

Class

Antimetabolite
Cell Cycle Specific

Indications

Acute leukemias, chronic myelocytic leukemia, lymphomas, as an immunosuppressant to prevent rejection of homografts

Dosages

Vary according to individual protocols.
Induction: 2.5 mg/kg day PO
   80–100 mg/m²/day PO
Maintenance: 50–100 mg/m²/day PO
   1.5–2.5 mg/kg/day PO

Reconstitution

None: 50-mg tablets

Administration

Oral

Stability

Check package for expiration date.
Store tablets at room temperature.

Side Effects

Anemia, anorexia, dermatologic reaction, flu-like reaction (fever, headache, weakness), **gastrointestinal alterations (diarrhea, nausea and vomiting), hepatic toxicity, leukopenia,** stomatitis, **thrombocytopenia**

Nurse Alert

- Patients who receive mercaptopurine and allopurinol concomitantly should have the dose of mercaptopurine reduced by 25%–33% because allopurinol inhibits the metabolism of oral mercaptopurine.
- Drug has been reported to both potentiate and diminish the anticoagulation activity of warfarin.

Mesna (Mesnex)

Class

Sulphydryl

Indications

Prophpylactic agent used to reduce the incidence of infostamide-induced hemorrhagic cystitis.

Dosages

Vary according to individual protocols.
Recommended dosage is 240 mh/m².
Mesna dose is 20% of Ifosfamide dose.

Reconstitution

Dilute with D_5W/NS to desired concentration.

Administration

IV 15 min before Ifosfamide
IV 4 and 8 hours after Ifosfamide

Stability

Reconstituted solution should be used within 6 hours.
Dilute solution is stable for 24 hours.

Side Effects

Nausea and vomiting, diarrhea

Nurse Alert

- Mesna prevents Ifosfamide-induced hemorrhagic cystitis. It does not prevent cystitis in all patients, so monitoring prior to each dose should be done (examine a morning specimen of urine for RBCs).
- Mesna does *not* prevent or alleviate other adverse reactions.

Methotrexate/A-Methopterin/MTX (Mexate, Folex)

Class

Antimetabolite
Cell Cycle Specific

Indication

Gestational choriocarcinoma, chorioadenoma destruens, hydatidiform moles, acute lymphocytic leukemia, breast carcinoma, epidermoid carcinoma of the head and neck, squamous cell and small cell carcinomas of the lung, lymphosarcomas, lymphomas, osteogenic sarcomas; prophylaxis and treatment of meningeal leukemia; advanced cases of mycosis fungoides, psoriasis, rheumatoid arthritis

Dosages

Vary according to individual protocols.
Leukemia: 3.3 mg/m^2 IV daily for 4–6 weeks
Choriocarcinomas: 15–30 mg IV daily × 5 days
Gastrointestinal tumors: 100–250 mg/m^2 IV
Osteogenic sarcomas (high dose): 8–12 gm/m^2 IV
Intrathecal treatments (weekly or twice weekly): 12 mg/m^2 or an empirical dose of 15 mg

Reconstitution

Liquid form (25 mg/cc) requires no mixing.

Dilute powder with D_5W, normal saline, or sterile water for injection at a concentration no greater than 25 mg/cc.

For intrathecal administration, dilute with a preservative-free medium of sodium chloride or Elliott's B Solution in a volume of 2–5 cc to decrease the incidence of subarachnoiditis.

Administration

PO, IM, IV, intrathecal, or intra-arterial

Stability

Check package for expiration date.

Ready-to-use vials are stable at room temperature.

Dilute powdered vials immediately prior to use.

Side Effects

Alopecia, anaphpylaxis, **anemia,** dermatologic reactions (photosensitivity, rash), **gastrointestinal alterations (abdominal distress, nausea, diarrhea, and vomiting),** hepatic toxicities, **leukopenia,** neurotoxicities (dizziness, **fatigue, headache),** renal toxicity (tubular necrosis), **stomatitis, thrombocytopenia,** pulmonary toxicity (pneumonias, cough, fever, eosinophilia, cyanosis)

(continued)

Methotrexate (continued)

Nurse Alert

- Normal BUN and creatinine levels must be present prior to administration of methotrexate.
- Use with extreme caution in patients with "third spacing" (e.g., ascites, pleural effusions, pedal edema), because the protein in this fluid binds with the methotrexate and does not allow for proper elimination of the drug, thereby enhancing the toxicities.
- For high-dose administration, adequate hydration with sodium bicarbonate and leucovorin rescue must be closely monitored to prevent life-threatening toxicities.
- Keep urine alkaline (a pH greater than 7), usually with allopurinol.
- Toxicities increase with concomitant administration of sulfanomides, sulfonylureas, phenytoin, salicylates, phenylbutazone, tetracycline, chloramphenicol, and para-aminobenzoic acid.
- Because of the incidence of photosensitivity, use sun blocks of SPF 15 or greater with any exposure to sunlight.
- Refer to leucovorin calcium, page 105, prior to administration of high-dose methotrexate.

Mitomycin (Mutamycin)

Class

Antineoplastic Antibiotic
Cell Cycle Nonspecific

Indications

Gastrointestinal, pancreatic, breast, lung,
cervical, bladder, head and neck, and
ovarian carcinomas; chronic myelogenous
leukemia

Dosages

2 mg/m^2 daily × 5 days, 2 days drug-free,
repeat course for a total initial dose of 20
mg/m^2 over 10 days
5–20 mg/m^2 IV every 6–8 weeks

Reconstitution

Add 10 cc sterile water to 5-mg vials
Add 40 cc sterile water to 20-mg vials
Yield: 0.5 mg/1 cc

Administration

IV push slowly via the side arm of a rapidly
running IV
Topical instillation (bladder)
Intra-arterial (colon)

(continued)

Mitomycin (continued)

Stability

Check package for expiration date.
Reconstituted drug is stable for 7 days at room temperature or 14 days when refrigerated.

Side Effects

Alopecia, anemia, anorexia, dermatologic reactions (skin rashes), extravasation, **fever,** gastrointestinal alterations (diarrhea, **nausea and vomiting), ** hepatic toxicities, **leukopenia, malaise, pulmonary toxicity (pulmonary fibrosis and interstitial pneumonitis), renal toxicities (increased BUN, creatinine), stomatitis, thrombocytopenia**

Nurse Alert

- Drug is a potent vesicant and peripheral administration must always be done in the constant attendance of an MD or an RN knowledgeable in chemotherapy. Never administer the drug if the IV site is compromised. (See chapter 3.)
- Thrombocytopenia may occur late and may be cumulative (4–8 weeks after treatment) and may last 2–3 weeks.

Mitotane (Lysodren)

Class

Miscellaneous
Mechanism of action unknown

Indications

Adrenocortical carcinoma

Dosages

Vary according to individual protocols.
2–16 gm/day in 3–4 divided doses
Dosages usually begin low and are titrated
  upward

Reconstitution

None: 500–mg tablets

Adminstration

Oral

Stability

Check package for expiration date.
Storage at room temperature.

(continued)

Mitotane (continued)

Side Effects

Anorexia, cardiac toxicity (orthostatic hypotension, hypertension, flushing), cystitis, dermatologic reaction (rash), fever, **gastrointestinal alterations (nausea, vomiting, diarrhea), neurotoxicity (somnolence, lethargy,** vertigo, headache, diplopia, retinopathy, lens opacities)

Nurse Alert

- Mitotane increases steriod metabolism, therefore larger than replacement doses of exogenous corticosteroids are required during therapy.
- Dose reduction/discontinuation may be warranted in presence of shock, trauma, or infection, because acute adrenal insufficiency may be precipitated by mitotane.
- Nausea/vomiting is a dose-limiting toxicity. Begin with a low dose and increase as tolerated.
- Excreted in urine.

Mitoxantrone (Novantrone)

Class

Anthracenediones-Antibiotic
Cell Cycle Specific

Indications

Non-lymphocytic leukemia

Dosages

Vary according to individual protocols.
10–14 mg/m²/day × 1–3 days

Reconstitution

Dilute in D_5W or NS

Stability

Stable at room temperature for 48 hours.

Administration

IV bolus

Side Effects

Allergic reaction, **alopecia, anemia, cardiotoxicity, leukopenia,** gastrointestinal alterations **(nausea and vomiting),** metabolic alterations (hyperuremia), mucositis, reproductive dysfunction, **thrombocytopenia**

(continued)

Mitoxantrone (continued)

Nurse Alert

- Incompatible with heparin.
- Patients urine may be blue-green for 24 hours after administration.
- Drug may act as a vesicant and peripheral administration should always be done in constant presence of an MD or RN knowledgeable in the administration of chemotherapy.

Paclitaxel (Taxol)

Class

Miscellaneous
Microtubule Promoter

Indications

Metastatic ovarian, breast, and lung cancer

Dosages

Vary according to individual protocols.
135–250 mg/m^2 every 3–4 weeks

Reconstitution

Dilute with bacteriostatic sterile water or NS
to a concentration of 0.3–1.2 mg/cc

Administration

Administer IV over 3, 24, or 96 hours.
Admix drug in glass bottles or polypropylene
bags. Non-PVC, polypropylene-lined
administration sets are recommended. In-
line 0.22 micron filters are necessary and
may require frequent (> q 24 hour) changing
due to clogging.

Stability

Check package insert for expiration date.
Vials must be refrigerated prior to use.
Reconstituted solution is stable for 24 hours.

(continued)

Paclitaxel (continued)

Side Effects

Leukopenia, anemia, thrombocytopenia, **hypersensitivity reaction, neurotoxicities (parethesias, myalgias, arthralgias) hepatotoxicity, cardiotoxicity (hypotension, asymptomatic bradycardia), alopecia,** gastrointestinal alterations (mucositis, nausea, diarrhea)

Nurse Alert

- **All patients must be pretreated for potential hypersensitivity reaction. Pretreatment includes steroids, Diphenhydramine, H_2 antagonist.** This reaction may be due to the drug or the Cremophor-L in which it is mixed. Usual pretreatment includes Dexamethasone 20 mh 6 and 12 hours prior to treatment and 50 mg Diphenhydramine with 300 mg Cimetidine or 50 mg Ranitidine 30 min prior to treatment.
- Controversy about whether to classify drug as a vesicant or an irritant exists.
- Administering long-term infusions via central line is recommended.
- Infiltrations are managed with heat.
- Side effects seem to be related to duration of infusions.

Plicamycin (Mithracin)

Class

Antibiotic
Cell Cycle Nonspecific
Inhibits Osteoclastic Activity

Indications

Testicular tumors, Paget's disease of the bone,
malignant hypercalcemia, glioblastoma
multiforme

Dosages

Vary according to individual protocols.
Testicular: 25–30 mcg/kg daily for 8–10 days
25–50 mcg/kg every other day × 8 days
Hypercalcemia: 25 mcg/kg IV × 1
25 mcg/kg IV × 3–4 days

Reconstitution

Add 4.9 cc of sterile water to 2.5-mg vial for
final concentration of 500 mcg/cc. May be
further diluted in D_5W or normal saline.

(continued)

Plicamycin (continued)

Administration

Drug is administered IV. Manufacturer recommends that the drug be administered over 4–6 hours to prevent/minimize nausea; however, drug is a vesicant and must be monitored constantly if administered peripherally. Consideration should be given to administration via a central line if the duration of administration is greater than 30 min.

Stability

Check package for expiration date.
Use reconstituted solution soon after mixing.
Refrigerate unreconstituted vials at 2°–8°C.

Side Effects

Alopecia, **anemia,** dermatologic reaction (facial flushing, papular excoriations, thickening of skin folds), fever, **gastrointestinal alterations** (diarrhea, **nausea, vomiting**), hepatic dysfunction (increased SGOT, LDH), leukopenia, metabolic alteration (decreased phosphate, magnesium, potassium, and calcium), neurotoxicity (headache, depression, irritability, **drowsiness**), renal toxicity (proteinurea, increased creatinine and BUN), **stomatitis, thrombocytopenia,** venous phlebitis

Nurse Alert

- Drug is a potent vesicant and peripheral administration must always be done in the constant attendance of an MD or an RN knowledgeable in chemotherapy. Never administer the drug if the IV site is compromised. (See chapter 3.)
- Coagulopathy can occur in up to 1/3 of patients receiving plicamycin; monitor prothrombin time, partial thromboplastin time, platelet counts, and obvious signs of bleeding.
- Contraindicated in patients with thrombocytopenia, thrombocoagulopathy, coagulation disorders, or any other disease associated with hemorrhage.
- Nausea and vomiting seem to decrease with a slower infusion of drug as opposed to IV bolus.
- Doses may be modified in patients with hypercalcemia associated with malignancy who may be receiving other chemotherapeutic agents to treat their primary cancer.
- Ordered in micrograms (mcg), not milligrams (mg).
- Use with extreme caution in patients with preexisting hepatic or renal impairment.

Prednisone (Deltasone)

Class

Glucocorticoid

Indications

Used as part of combination chemotherapy for Hodgkin's disease, breast cancer lymphoma, and acute leukemia

Dosages

Vary according to individual protocols.
3–6 mg PO every day

Reconstitution

None: 1-, 5-, 10-, 20-, 50-mg tablets

Administration

Oral

Stability

See package for expiration date.

Side Effects

Cardiac toxicity (CHF, hypertension), **cushingoid appearance,** dermatologic toxicity (impaired healing, erythema, petechiae), gastrointestinal alterations (peptic ulcer, pancreatitis, abdominal distension, ulcerative esophagitis), latent diabetes mellitus, metabolic alterations (fluid retention, hypernatremia, hypokalemia, negative nitrogen balance), neurotoxicity (increased intracranial pressure, headache, confusion, vertigo, increased intraocular pressure), reproductive dysfunction (menstrual irregularities)

Nurse Alert

- Patients maintained on insulin or oral hypoglycemic agents may need to increase the doses of these medications.
- Take drug with milk or antacid to prevent gastrointestinal toxicity.

Procarbazine (Matulane)

Class

Miscellaneous
Cell Cycle Nonspecific

Indications

Hodgkin's and non-Hodgkin's lymphomas,
bronchogenic cancer, intracranial neoplasms

Dosages

100 mg/m² daily × 1 week increased to
150–200 mg/m² as tolerated for up to 3
weeks

Reconstitution

None: 50-mg capsules

Administration

Oral

Stability

Check package for expiration date.
Store at room temperature.

Side Effects

Anemia, arthralgias, **leukopenia,** neurotoxicity
(lethargy, drowsiness, peripheral neuropa-
thy, convulsions), dysphagia, **dermatologic**

reactions (rash, hyperpigmentation), gastro-intestinal alterations (diarrhea, **nausea and vomiting**), headache, hypotension, reproductive dysfunction (azoospermia, cessation of menses), secondary malignancies, stomatitis, **thrombocytopenia,** vertigo

Nurse Alert

- Drug is a monoamine oxidase inhibitor (MAO) and has Antabuse-like activity. It interacts and should not be taken with: alcohol, central nervous system depressants, hypoglycemic agents, levodopa, meperidine, sympathomimetic amines, tricyclic antidepressants, hypotensive agents, phenothiazines, and foods containing high amounts of tyramine (wine, cheese, beer, brewer's yeast, yogurt, pickled herring, chicken livers, and bananas).
- Causes delayed bone-marrow depression (2–5 weeks after treatment)

Streptozocin (Zanosar)

Class

Nitrosourea
Cell Cycle Nonspecific

Indications

Malignant carcinoid syndrome, Hodgkin's
disease, Zollinger-Ellison syndrome, colon,
liver, and pancreatic carcinomas

Dosages

500–1,500 mg/m^2 IV weekly
500 mg/m^2 IV daily × 5 days every 3–6 weeks

Reconstitution

Add 9.5 cc D$_5$W or normal saline for injection
to each 1-gm vial
Yield: 100 mg/1 cc
Dilute with an additional 100–250 cc normal
saline

Administration

Administer slowly IV.
Can also be administered via hepatic artery
continuous infusion.

Stability

Check package for expiration date.

After reconstitution, the drug is stable for 48 hours at room temperature or 96 hours under refrigeration; however, as the solution contains no preservative, it is recommended that any unused portion be discarded after 8 hours.

Side Effects

Anemia, gastrointestinal alterations (nausea and vomiting, diarrhea, abdominal cramps), **hepatic toxicities (mild elevation in SGOT, SGPT),** hypoglycemia, **leukopenia, renal toxicities** (proteinuria, increased BUN, creatinine), stomatitis, fluid retention, **thrombocytopenia**

Nurse Alert

- Drug is an irritant and should be diluted adequately to avoid any burning at the IV site; apply ice packs to alleviate some of the local discomfort.
- Almost all patients experience some nausea and vomiting. Administer antiemetic therapy prior to initiation of therapy.
- Monitor renal function (e.g., urine protein, serum creatinine, BUN levels).

Tamoxifen (Nolvadex)

Class

Antiestrogen

Indications

Breast cancer (usually estrogen-receptor positive), prostate cancer (investigational)

Dosages

10–20 mg twice a day

Reconstitution

None: 10-mg tablets

Administration

Oral

Stability

Check package for expiration date.
Store at room temperature.

Side Effects

Dermatologic reactions (skin rash), fluid retention, gastrointestinal alterations **(nausea, vomiting),** leukopenia, **metabolic alteration (hypercalcemia),** neurotoxicity (headache, dizziness, depression), pain (bone and tumor), **reproductive dysfunction (hot flashes, menstrual irregularities),** retinopathy, thrombocytopenia, **vaginal bleeding, vaginal discharge,** pruritus vulvae, venous phlebitis

Nurse Alert
- Some patients may experience a "flare" of their symptoms, especially bone and/or tumor pain.
- Medicate with analgesics until pain subsides. If the flare occurs after the first month of therapy, this is most likely disease progression.
- Premenopausal women must be counselled about birth control as tamoxifen can induce ovulation.
- Skin rash usually responds to topical steroids.

Thioguanine/6TG
(Thioguanine Tabloid)

Class

Antimetabolite
Cell Cycle Specific

Indications

Acute nonlymphocytic, lymphocytic, and
chronic myelocytic leukemia

Dosages

100 mg/m^2 every 12 hours × 5–10 days PO
2 mg/kg PO daily until toxicities occur

Reconstitution

None: 40-mg tablets

Administration

Oral
IV use is currently under investigation.

Stability

Check package for expiration date.
Refrigerate IV solution to avoid precipitation.

Side Effects

Anemia, anorexia, dermatologic reactions (rash), **hepatic veno-occlusive disease,** jaundice, **gastrointestinal alterations** (diarrhea, **nausea and vomiting), leukopenia,** photosensitivity, stomatitis, **thrombocytopenia**

Nurse Alert

- Allopurinol can be used in full doses with thioguanine (unlike mercaptopurine).
- Reduce dose with impaired liver or renal function.
- Give between meals to facilitate absorption.

Thiotepa (Thio-TEPA)

Class

Alkylating Agent
Cell Cycle Nonspecific

Indications

Bladder, breast, ovarian cancer; Hodgkin's
disease; leptomeningeal cancer; intracavitary metastatic effusions

Dosages

Vary according to individual protocols.
Bladder: Instill 60 mg/60 cc sterile water every
week
Intracavitary: 30–60 mg/m^2 every week
Parenteral: 6–8 mg/m^2 IV × 5 days every 2–4
weeks
10–30 mg/m^2 IV every week
15–60 mg IM/subcutaneously every week
Intrathecal: 1–10 mg/m^2

Reconstitution

Dilute 15-mg vial with 1.5 cc sterile water for
injection for final concentration of 10 mg/cc.
For intrathecal use dilute with 15 cc of
preservative-free sterile water for injection
for final concentration of 1 mg/cc. If mixed
with Elliott's B Solution, the resulting
hypertonic mix may injure the spinal
column.

For intracavitary use drug may be further
diluted; use 10–20 cc isotonic saline for
intrapleural/pericardial instillation; 60 cc of
sterile water for bladder instillation.

Administration
IV push, IM, intramuscularly, intracavitary,
intrathecally, or directly into the tumor

Stability
Check package for expiration date.
Store unreconstituted powder in refrigerator.
Reconstituted solution is stable for 5 days
under refrigeration.

Side Effects
Allergic reaction (hives, bronchoconstriction),
anemia, **anorexia**, fever, **gastrointestinal
alterations (nausea, vomiting), leukopenia,**
neurotoxicities (headache, dizziness),
reproductive dysfunction (amenorrhea,
interference with spermatogenesis),
thrombocytopenia

(continued)

Thiotepa (continued)

Nurse Alert

- Bladder instillation: Instill via Foley catheter and retain for 2 hours; have patient change position every 15 min.
- Modify doses for patients with hepatic, renal, or bone-marrow dysfunction.
- Severity of bone-marrow depression is increased when thiotepa is given with radiation therapy and/or other alkylating agents.
- Weeping or breakdown from a subcutaneous lesion may occur when drug is instilled directly into tumor.

Vinblastine (Velban)

Class
Vinca Alkaloid
Cell Cycle Specific

Indications
Hodgkin's and non-Hodgkin's lymphomas,
Kaposi's sarcoma, gestational choriocarcinomas, mycosis fungoides, neuroblastomas,
testicular, head and neck, breast and renal
carcinomas

Dosages
5–6 mg/m^2 IV every 1–3 weeks
5.5–7.4 mg/m^2 IV weekly

Reconstitution
Add 10 cc normal saline to 10-mg vial
Yield: 1 mg/1 cc

Administration
IV push slowly via the side arm of a rapidly
running IV
Investigational: long-term IV infusion

(continued)

Vinblastine (continued)

Stability

Check package for expiration date.
Vials must be stored under refrigeration.
Reconstituted solution is stable for 30 days
under refrigeration when protected from
light.

Side Effects

Alopecia, **anemia,** dermatologic reactions
(rash), extravasation, **gastrointestinal alterations** (constipation, diarrhea, abdominal
pain in high doses, **nausea and vomiting),
leukopenia,** neurotoxicities (headache,
peripheral neuropathies, photosensitivity,
mental depression), stomatitis,
thrombocytopenia

Nurse Alert

- Drug is a potent vesicant and peripheral
  administration must always be done in the
  constant attendance of an MD or an RN
  knowledgeable in chemotherapy. Never
  administer the drug if the IV site is
  compromised. (See chapter 3.)
- Prophylactic stool softeners may be helpful
  in combating constipation.

Vincristine (Oncovin, Vincosar)

Class

Vinca Alkaloid
Cell Cycle Specific

Indications

Acute leukemia, non-Hodgkin's lymphoma,
Hodgkin's disease, Wilms' tumor, Ewing's
sarcoma, neuroblastoma, rhabdomyosarcoma,
refractory idiopathic thrombocytopenia
purpura, brain, breast, cervix, lung cancer

Dosages

Vary according to individual protocols.
0.4–1.4 mg/m^2 IV every week
Single dose not to exceed 2.0 mg

Reconstitution

Liquid form (1 mg/cc) requires no mixing.
Nonreconstituted 1-mg and 5-mg vials come
with their own 10-cc diluent. When reconstituted, the final concentration is
    1-mg vial = 0.1 mg/cc
    5-mg vial = 0.5 mg/cc

Administration

IV push through side arm of rapidly running IV

(continued)

Vincristine (continued)

Stability

Check package for expiration date.
Refrigerate vials/syringes.
Reconstituted vials are stable for up to 15 days
under refrigeration.
Protect from light.

Side Effects

**Alopecia, gastrointestinal alterations (consti-
pation),** leukopenia, metabolic alterations
(hyponatremia) **neurotoxicities (numbness,
weakness, paresthesias, ataxia, ptosis, foot
drop, jaw pain, decreased deep tendon
reflexes, slapping gait, mental depression)**

Nurse Alert

- Drug is a potent vesicant and peripheral
  administration must always be done in the
  constant attendance of an MD or RN knowledge in chemotherapy. Never administer the
  drug if the IV site is compromised. (See
  chapter 3.)
- Recommended antidote for extravasation is
  hyaluronidase (See chapter 3.)
- Prophylactic bowel regimen may be utilized
  to decrease chance of constipation.
- Dose modifications are needed in patients
  with liver disease.

- Older patients seem more sensitive to neurotoxicities.
- Reversal of neurotoxicities can take months after drug is discontinued.

Vindesine (Eldisine, Desacetylrinblastine)

Class

Synthetic Vinca Alkaloid
Cell Cycle Specific

Indications

Same as Velban

Dosages

Vary according to individual protocols.
3–4 mg/m^2 every 1–2 weeks
1–1.3 mg/m^2/day × 5–7 days every 21 days
1.5–2 mg/m^2 twice a week

Reconstitution

Mix 10-mg vial with provided diluent or NS.

Administration

Slow IV push
Continuous IV infusion

Stability

Check package for expiration date.
After reconstitution the solution is stable for 3
weeks if refrigerated.

Side Effects

Myelosuppession, neuropathies, alopecia,
anemia, anorexia, gastrointestinal alteration
**(constipation, nausea and vomiting),
leukopenia,** stomatitis, thrombocytopenia

Nurse Alert

- Drug is potent vesicant and peripheral administration should always be done in the constant attendance of an MD or an RN knowledgeable in the administration of chemotherapy.
- Recommended antidote for extravasation is hyaluronidase.
- Do not give with other vinca alkaloids as neurotoxicity could be cumulative.
- Dose reduction is necessary with abnormal LFTs.

Vinorelbine (Navelbine)

Class

Vinca Alkaloid
Cell Cycle Specific

Indications

Non-small cell lung cancer

Dosages

Vary according to individual protocols.
30 mg/m^2 IV every week

Reconstitution

Dilute in syringe or IV solution using D$_5$W or
NS

Syringe: dilute to concentration of 1.5 and 3.0
mg/cc

IV bag: dilute to concentration between 0.5
and 2.0 mg/cc

Administration

IV through side arm of rapidly running IV.
Flush with 75–125 cc of NS or D$_5$W

Stability

Check package insert for expiration date.
Store unopened vials in refrigerator. If stored
at room temperature, stability is 72 hours.
Diluted drug is stable for 24 hours at room
temperature.

Side Effects

> **Leukopenia,** anemia, gastrointestinal alterations (constipation, **nausea,** vomiting, diarrhea), peripheral neuropathy, **integumentary (injection site reactions,** alopecia), fatigue, dyspnea

Nurse Alert

- Drug is a vesicant and peripheral administration must always be done in the attendance of an MD or RN knowledgeable in chemotherapy. Never administer the drug if the IV site is compromised. (See chapter 3.)
- Treat extravasation same as for other vinca alkaloids.
- Injection-site reaction may occur after 12 doses of Navelbine. This may occur locally or along the length of the vein.

V

Nursing Management & Patient Education Regarding Side Effects

Alopecia

Patients at Risk

- Receiving Actinomycin D, Bleomycin, Cyclophosphamide*, Cytosine Arabinoside, Daunorubicin*, Doxorubicin*, Fluorouracil, Hexamethylmelamine, Hydroxyurea, Idarubicin*, Ifosfamide, Lomustine, Methotrexate, Mitomycin C, Mitroxantrone, Nitrogen Mustard, Paclitaxel, Semustine, Streptozocin, Vinblastine, Vincristine*, Vindesine, VM-26, VP-16.
- Receiving whole brain radiation therapy

Assessment

- Hair thinning or loss (head or body hair)

Possible Nursing Diagnosis

- Disturbance in self-concept: body image

Nursing Actions

- Reassure that hair will grow back; new hair growth usually occurs about 8 weeks after completion of the chemotherapy; the new hair is usually coarser.
- Refer to American Cancer Society or Social Service Department if finances for a wig are a problem.

---

*High incidence

Patient Teaching

- Inform of potential hair loss and encourage to purchase hairpiece prior to actual hair loss to assure natural fit and style.
- Encourage to check insurance policy for possible reimbursement. Some policies will reimburse if patient presents prescription for "cranial prosthesis" or "medically induced hair prosthesis." A wig is a tax-deductible medical expense.
- Alert to possible loss of body hair as well as scalp hair. Eyebrow pencil and makeup can help minimize the change in appearance.
- Discourage from using harsh chemicals (hair dyes, sprays, permanents) during treatments.
- Teach to protect scalps during times of alopecia (e.g., wear hats, scarves, wigs when out of doors).
- Instruct to use a mild non-alcohol-based lotion (e.g., pure lanolin, Keri lotion) if scalp burning and itching occurs.

Allergic Reactions/Anaphylaxis

Patients at Risk

- Receiving Amsacrine, Asparaginase*, Bleo-mycin*, Cyclophosphamide, Daunorubicin, Doxorubicin, Etoposide, Mechlorethamine, Melphalan, Methotrexate, Paclitaxel, Platinol*, Procarbazine, VM-26

Assessment

Note: Incidence of anaphylaxis usually increases with continued exposure to drug.

- Itching
- Flushing of the skin
- Dizziness
- Chills
- Respiratory distress
- Chest or throat discomfort/tightness
- "Anything unusual"

Possible Nursing Diagnoses

- Ineffective airway clearance
- Ineffective breathing pattern
- Impaired gas exchange
- Impaired skin integrity
- Alteration in comfort (pruritus)

Nursing Actions

- Obtain allergy history and document on patient record.

---

*High incidence

- Obtain baseline vital signs before chemotherapy.
- Perform skin testing and/or test dose prior to administration of drugs with high incidence of allergic reaction (e.g., asparaginase, bleomycin in lymphoma patients).
- Have emergency equipment available and labeled for immediate use.
- Have epinephrine, diphenhydramine (Benadryl), and hydrocortisone at bedside.
- Ensure MD is present during administration of asparaginase.
- Obtain order for premedication (diphenhydramine and/or hydrocortisone) for asparaginase.
- If allergic reaction is suspected
  - discontinue the chemotherapy,
  - infuse normal saline or D_5W to maintain open line,
  - quickly assess for localized versus generalized reaction.

Localized
- *Signs and symptoms:* erythema at site of chemotherapy administration, urticaria, wheals, burning, itching
- *Treatment:* diphenhydramine and/or hydrocortisone; monitor vital signs; observe injection site.

(continued)

Allergic Reactions (continued)

- Cautiously proceed with chemotherapy after medication and in the presence of an MD; have emergency cart available; monitor patient for further allergic episodes.

Generalized
- *Signs and symptoms:* itching, chest discomfort, respiratory distress, hypotension, cramping, facial edema, urticaria, nausea, cyanosis, agitation, fear
- *Treatment:*
  - call for emergency help
  - infuse maintenance IV at rate necessary to maintain blood pressure
  - monitor vital signs every 2–5 min
  - if hypotensive, elevate patient's feet
  - maintain airway
  - administer oxygen at 2 l/min via nasal prongs
  - Medications
    + epinephrine 1:1,000 (0.3–0.75 cc IV)
    + diphenhydramine (50 mg IM)
    + hydrocortisone (0.5 mg–1 mg/kg IV)
    + aminophylline (doses dependent on age and size of patient and activity of allergic response)

Patient Teaching
- Provide with a list of names of medications to which patient is allergic.
- Provide with information regarding Medic-Alert bracelets/cards.
- List signs and symptoms of allergic reaction and the importance of reporting them immediately to RN, MD.

Anemia

Patients at Risk

- Receiving chemotherapy drugs that suppress the bone marrow (most agents)
- With nutritional deficiencies
- With hematologic malignancies
- With solid tumors metastatic to the bone marrow
- Receiving prior and/or concomitant radiation therapy
- Who have undergone surgery, especially splenectomy, gastrectomy, colon resection

Assessment

- Fatigue
- Shortness of breath
- Tachycardia
- Dizziness; ringing in the ears
- Pallor
- Headache
- Obvious sites of bleeding (stool, urine, sputum, oral cavity)
- Pertinent lab values: Hct/Hgb, WBC, platelet count, vitamin B_{12}/folic acid (when appropriate), iron, total iron binding capacity (when appropriate)

Possible Nursing Diagnoses

- Activity intolerance
- Impaired gas exchange

Nursing Actions

- Obtain dietary consult regarding iron-rich foods.
- Give iron supplements as ordered; inform of constipating effects of iron and darkening of stools.
- Assess hydration status, since hematocrit is increased in dehydrated patients and anemia may not be diagnosed until patient is rehydrated.
- Promote rest; prioritize activities and tests.
- Provide blankets and socks for warmth as patients may complain of being cold.
- Institute safety precautions if patient is dizzy or lightheaded.
- Administer pharmocologic agents such as recombinant human erythopoietin which stimulate the erythopoietic response.
- Administer blood transfusions; observe for transfusion reaction, fluid overload.
- Administer oxygen therapy if patient is short of breath (usually not seen until Hgb falls below 8.0/gm/dl).

Patient Teaching

- Teach signs and symptoms of anemia.
- Caution to adjust lifestyle to include rest periods during times of bone-marrow suppression.

(continued)

Anemia (continued)

- Discuss the importance of nutritionally balanced diet.
- Warn about the possibility of constipating effects of iron supplements and the resulting dark stools.

Anorexia

Patients at Risk

- Receiving chemotherapy (any type)
- With metastatic disease
- Suffering from nausea, stomatitis, taste changes, depression, constipation, pain
- On pain medication
- Receiving chemotherapy likely to cause taste changes
  - Carboplatin
  - Cisplatin
  - Cytoxan
  - DTIC
  - Mechlorethamine
  - Fluorouracil
  - Methotrexate

Assessment

- Weight loss
- Lack of interest in food
- Poor skin turgor
- Complaints of taste changes (e.g., decreased threshold for bitterness; increased threshold for sweets; aversion to sweets, red meat, coffee; metallic taste in mouth)
- Pertinent lab values: serum albumin, CBC, electrolytes

(continued)

Anorexia (continued)

Possible Nursing Diagnoses

- Alteration in nutrition: less than body requirements
- Sensory-perceptual alteration: gustatory

Nursing Actions

- Obtain baseline height/weight.
- Weigh each visit when outpatient; weigh twice a week when in hospital.
- Obtain a dietary consult for calculation of nutritional requirements, recommendations for supplements and calorie count.
- Obtain dietary history regarding food preferences, taste changes, allergies. (Patients with a lactose intolerance can drink lactose-free milk or some "fast food" shakes, which contain no milk products.)
- Medicate with antiemetics before meals if nausea is a problem.
- Give appetite stimulants as ordered (e.g., steroids, periactin, megace).
- Manage symptoms of pain, constipation, stomatitis, depression.

Patient Teaching

- Eat smaller, more frequent meals.
- Drink wine as an aperitif with meals (in moderation and after checking with the MD).

- Increase calories by adding gravies, sauces, cream, etc.
- Increase protein intake with milk, cheeses, yogurt, legumes, poultry, fish.
- Use nutritional supplements (Ensure, Sustacal, Meritene, Carnation Instant Breakfast, milkshakes, eggnog, yogurt).
- Avoid fluids before meals because they can create a sense of fullness.
- Avoid foods with strong odors.
- Offer foods at room temperature (usually better tolerated).
- Practice good oral hygiene.
- Use oral anesthetics cautiously prior to meals as gag reflect may be affected.
- Provide meal preparer with written material on nutrition (available from American Cancer Society, National Cancer Institute, private drug companies).
- Try to change environment for meals (e.g., get out of bed when possible).
- Exercise prior to meals.
- Experiment with different spices if taste alterations occur; use spices cautiously if stomatitis is a problem.

Cardiac Toxicity

Patients at Risk

- Patients receiving Dactinomycin*, Daunomycin*, Doxorubicin*, Cytoxan (high dose),
  Epirubicin*, Estrogens, Paclitaxel

Assessment

- Dry cough
- Dyspnea
- Rales
- Tachycardia
- Distended neck veins
- Pedal edema
- ECG changes: ST-T wave changes,
  diminished QRS complex, PVCs
- Cardiomegaly
- Hepatomegaly
- Decreased cardiac ejection fraction
- Pertinent lab values: CBC (low Hgb/Hct can
  present with some symptoms of cardio-
  toxicity), cardiac ejection fraction, potas-
  sium level (especially if on duretics),
  echocardiogram, serial ECGs

---

*Cardiac toxicity appears to be dose-dependent, with
the risk increasing proportionally to cumulative
dosages. It is very important that accurate documenta-
tion of cumulative drug dosages is maintained. Maximum doses: daunorubicin 600 mg/m^2, doxorubucin
550 mg/m^2, epirubicin 1,100 mg/m^2.

Possible Nursing Diagnoses
- Alteration in cardiac output: decreased
- Activity intolerance

Nursing Actions
- Monitor vital signs every 2–4 hours.
- Administer inotropic drugs as ordered by MD to increase cardiac output.
- Administer O_2 for respiratory comfort as needed.
- Administer diuretics.
- Weigh every day.
- Monitor intake and output.
- Consult with coronary care nurses for treatment geared towards symptom relief and decreased cardiac-related morbidity.

Patient Teaching
- Teach signs and symptoms of cardiac toxicity.
- Discuss modifications/restricted diet if necessary.
- Help plan activity modifications as needed.

Constipation

Patients at Risk

- Receiving potentially neurotoxic chemotherapy (e.g., vinca alkaloids), Vindesine
- Receiving analgesics
- With underlying gastrointestinal disease
- With anorexia
- With hypercalcemia
- With spinal cord compression
- Demonstrating signs of mental changes or stress

Assessment

- Absence of bowel movement for 3 or more days
- Absence of bowel sounds
- Abdominal distension and pain
- Anorexia
- Nausea and vomiting
- Frequent watery stools
- Pertinent lab values: electrolytes, calcium

Possible Nursing Diagnosis

- Alteration in bowel elimination: constipation

Nursing Actions

- Monitor bowel habits:
  - frequency,
  - color,

- consistency,
- use of laxatives and stool softeners,
- dietary habits.
- Maintain accurate bowel movement record.
- Auscultate abdomen for bowel sounds (baseline and every shift until constipation resolved).
- Assess food and fluid intake
  - encourage increase in dietary fiber
  - encourage fluid intake to 2,000 cc/day unless contraindicated
- Encourage moderate exercise as tolerated.
- Administer laxatives and stool softeners as ordered, especially if patient is receiving narcotics regularly.
- Perform manual disimpaction and administer enemas only if CBC is within normal range.

Patient Teaching

- Teach signs and symptoms of constipation.
- Explain importance of maintaining balance of exercise and rest.
- Teach importance of maintaining adequate fluid intake.
- Caution about potential hazards of self-medication for constipation.

Cystitis

Patients at Risk

- Receiving Cyclophosphamide, Doxorubicin (if administered after cyclophosphamide), Hexamethylmelamine
- Who are dehydrated
- Who are predisposed to bladder or kidney dysfunction

Assessment

- Increase in the frequency/urgency of urination
- Dysuria
- Hematuria
- Low back pain
- Pertinent lab values: urinalysis, CBC

Possible Nursing Diagnoses

- Alteration in patterns of urinary elimination
- Alteration in comfort: pain

Nursing Actions

- Obtain urine for analysis and culture.
- Hematest all urine specimens.
- Monitor intake and output.
- Ensure fluid intake to maintain urine pH at less than or equal to 7.0.

- Administer antispasmodics as ordered:
  - phenazopyridine (Pyridium); urine turns orange
  - flavoxate HCI (Urispas)
  - ethoxazene HCI (Serenium)
- For severe cases of cystitis
  - Irrigate bladder as ordered.
  - Provide IV hydration.
  - Insert Foley catheter (caution with low WBC).

Patient Teaching

- Reinforce that prevention is key; drink at least 3 liters of fluid a day during chemotherapy.
- Void at onset of urge and before going to bed.
- Take oral cyclophosphamide early in the day to prevent drug remaining in the bladder overnight.
- Teach signs and symptoms of cystitis.
- Avoid coffee, tea, alcohol, and spices, which can further irritate bladder epithelium.

Dermatologic Reactions

Radiation Recall

Patients at Risk

- Receiving Actinomycin D, Bleomycin, Cyclophosphamide, Doxorubicin, 5-Fluorouracil, Hydroxyurea, Methotrexate, Vinblastine, Vincristine
- Receiving radiation therapy

Assessment

- A rash occurring at the site of radiation therapy when the radiation therapy is given concomitantly or prior to chemotherapy.

Possible Nursing Diagnosis

- Impaired skin integrity

Nursing Actions

Dry Reaction with Erythema
- Use mild soap and soft cloth when cleansing skin.
- Apply cortisone cream to relieve itching.

Wet Desquamation
- Culture drainage.
- Irrigate area with ½ strength H_2O_2 and rinse with normal saline; allow air to dry.
- Apply bio-occlusive dressing; do not use tape over area.

Patient Teaching
- Keep area free of clothes that rub; wear all-cotton material over area.
- Do not use heat on area (heating pads, compresses, etc.).
- Do not scratch skin.

Photosensitivity
Patients at Risk
- Receiving Actinomycin D, Bleomycin, Dacarbazine, Doxorubicin, Fluorouracil, Methotrexate, Vinblastine
- With a known sensitivity to the sun

Assessment
- Profound sunburn after minimal exposure to the sun
- Complaints of eyes burning/hurting with light

Possible Nursing Diagnoses
- Impaired skin integrity
- Sensory-perceptual alteration: vision
- Alteration in comfort
- Potential for infection

Nursing Actions
- Treat as a burn with cooling lotions (non-alcohol or non-perfume-based) and baths
- Use pain-management techniques as needed.
- Protect from infection.
- Keep exposed to air.

(continued)

Dermatologic Reactions (continued)

Patient Teaching

- Sunburn can occur with minimal exposure.
- Protect exposed areas of skin (e.g., wear hats, socks, long-sleeved shirts).
- Use sunscreen with SPF greater than 15 when outdoors.
- Minimize time spent in the sun.
- Wear dark glasses if light hurts eyes.
- Keep room darkened.

Urticaria/Erythema

Patients at Risk

- Receiving Bleomycin, Doxorubicin, L-Asparaginase, Mechlorethamine, Plicamycin

Assessment

- Generalized or localized redness along the venous route of chemotherapy

Possible Nursing Diagnoses

- Impaired skin integrity
- Potential for injury (anaphylaxis)

Nursing Actions

- In the presence of urticaria, monitor patient after L-Asparaginase for the development of a more serious hypersensitvity reaction; skin test prior to administering this drug again. (Refer to Allergic Reactions/ Anaphylaxis, pages 164–167.)

- Know that usually this condition is self-limiting within a few hours, but in severe cases chemotherapy may need to be discontinued.

Patient Teaching
- Tell/notify RN immediately if shortness of breath develops or the severity of the urticaria increases.
- Explain that urticaria is usually self-limiting and is not a cause of concern.

Hyperpigmentation
Patients at Risk
- Receiving Bleomycin, Busulfan, Carmustine, Cyclophosphamide, Daunorubicin, Doxorubicin, 5-Fluorouracil, Methotrexate

Assessment
- Darkening of the nail beds, mucous membranes, skin over joints, teeth, or venous route

Possible Nursing Diagnosis
- Disturbance in self-concept: body image

Nursing Actions/Patient Teaching
- Explain that the hyperpigmentation reaction will gradually subside 3–4 months post-treatment.

Diarrhea

Patients at Risk
- Receiving any chemotherapy (particularly 5-Fluorouracil)
- Receiving radiation therapy to abdomen or pelvis
- Receiving antibiotic therapy
- With tumors of the gastrointestinal tract
- Experiencing stress
- With a fecal impaction
- Receiving supplemental feedings

Assessment
- Abdominal cramping and bloating
- Loose, watery stools
- Weight loss
- Hyperactive bowel sounds
- Pertinent lab values· electrolytes, especially potassium

Possible Nursing Diagnoses
- Alteration in bowel elimination: diarrhea
- Fluid volume deficit
- Alteration in comfort: pain
- Impaired skin integrity (perianal)

Nursing Actions
- Monitor bowel habits:
  - frequency,
  - color,

- consistency,
- use of laxatives and stool softeners,
- dietary habits.
- Maintain accurate bowel movement record.
- Auscultate abdomen for bowel sounds.
- Assess food and fluid intake; encourage fluid intake to greater than or equal to 3,000 cc/day unless contraindicated.
- Question regarding lactose intolerance.
- Order diet low in residue but high in calories and protein.
- Avoid foods/beverages containing caffeine.
- Assess sources of psychologic stress and make appropriate referrals.
- Administer antidiarrhea medication as ordered.
- Assess socioeconomic factors that may affect maintenance of a well-balanced diet.
- Encourage rest and relaxed activity.
- Perform good perianal or ostomy care.
  - Wash area with mild soap and water after each bowel movement.
  - If perianal area is irritated:
    + apply A & D ointment,
    + use topical anesthetics as needed,
    + take sitz baths with solution of 1 liter normal saline, 40 gm $NaHCO_3$, 120 ml diphenhydramine elixir, and 120 ml viscous lidocaine.

(continued)

Diarrhea (continued)

Patient Teaching

- Teach good perineal or ostomy care.
- Instruct how to administer antidiarrhea medications, take sitz baths.
- Discuss dietary modifications for low-residue, high-calorie, high-protein diet.

Flu-like Syndrome

Patients at Risk

- Those receiving Bleomycin, Interferon

Assessment

- Pertinent lab values: WBC (to check if symptoms could be due to leukopenia-induced sepsis)
- Chills
- Fever
- Muscle ache
- Headache

Possible Nursing Diagnoses

- Alteration in comfort
- Hyperthermia

Nursing Actions

- Stop infusion of chemotherapy.
- Monitor temperature, vital signs.
- If symptoms subside, chemotherapy may be restarted in conjunction with acetaminophen and diphenhydramine as ordered.
- Be aware that flu-like symptoms may progress to anaphylaxis in lymphoma patients receiving bleomycin; give a test dose of bleomycin prior to the initiation of full-dose therapy.

(continued)

Flu-like Syndrome (continued)

Patient Teaching

- Tell patients that flu-like symptoms usually occur 2–10 hours after chemotherapy is administered.
- Advise that severity of symptoms usually decreases with successive doses.

Hepatic Toxicity

Patients at Risk

- Receiving Asparaginase, Cytarabine, Dacarbazine, Doxorubicin, Etoposide, Methotrexate, Mitomycin, Streptozocin, Thioguanine
- With impaired liver function, disease, or metastasis

Assessment

- Jaundice (skin, sclera)
- Light- or clay-colored stools
- Dark amber urine
- Liver enlargement (hepatomegaly) or tenderness
- Increased abdominal girth
- Impaired mental status (lethargy, confusion, disorientation)
- Asterixis
- Nausea/anorexia
- Pruritus
- Pertinent lab values: LDH, SGOT, SGPT, alkaline phosphatase, bilirubin, clotting studies

Possible Nursing Diagnoses

- Alteration in nutrition: less than body requirements
- Fluid volume excess
- Alteration in comfort
- Impaired skin integrity
- Altered thought processes

(continued)

Hepatic Toxicity (continued)

Nursing Actions

- Hold chemotherapy as ordered until resolution of hepatic toxicity.
- Measure abdominal girth, weigh each day.
- Institute safety precautions if mentally impaired.
- Medicate for nausea as needed.
- Provide nutritional support if anorexia is profound. (Refer to Anorexia, pages 171–173.)
- Keep skin lubricated with water-based moisturizer if pruritus present.

Patient Teaching

- List signs and symptoms of hepatic toxicity and importance of reporting them immediately to physician.
- Avoid alcohol.

Leukopenia

Patients at Risk

- Receiving chemotherapy (all types); see table 5.1.
- Receiving radiation therapy
- With bone-marrow involvement

Assessment

- Integumentary system (e.g., skin folds, wounds, catheter sites, body cavities): redness, pain, edema, or discharge (discharge may not be purulent due to abnormally low WBC)
- Respiratory system: cough, sore throat, sputum, shortness of breath, pleuritic pain
- Genitourinary system: dysuria, frequency, urgency, change in color or odor of urine
- Fever greater than 100°F, generalized aches, myalgias
- Pertinent lab values: WBC with differential, reticulocyte count, Hct/Hgb, platelet count

Possible Nursing Diagnoses

- Potential for infection
- Activity intolerance

Nursing Actions

- Take vital signs every 4 hours.
- Avoid rectal temperatures, enemas, and medications.

(continued)

Leukopenia (continued)

- Avoid catheterizations.
- Encourage coughing and deep breathing and use incentive spirometer regularly.
- Institute oral hygiene program: clean with baking soda and water every 2 hours, daily oral assessment.
- Perform good perineal care: use stool softener, cleanse well after each bowel movement, prevent rectal trauma.
- Change IV tubing and dressings daily.
- Perform all dressing changes and procedures utilizing sterile technique.
- Utilize good handwashing and aseptic technique; alter environment to minimize risk of infection.
- Institute reverse isolation when WBC is less than 1,000 mm^3.
- Ensure proper staffing to avoid cross-contamination with other patients.
- Prevent pressure sores by turning and repositioning every 2 hours.
- Administer pharmocologic agents such as colony stimulating factors that stimulate the proliferation of blood cells.

Patient Teaching

- List signs and symptoms of infection.
- Teach good sexual hygiene (urinate before/after sex, avoid oral sex, avoid douching and tampons while WBC is less than 1,000 mm^3.)
- Avoid plants and flowers (possible carriers of pseudomonas); avoid stagnant water (e.g., soap dishes, plants).
- Wash all fresh fruits and vegetables.
- Avoid elective surgery and dental work.

Table 5.1
Myelosuppressive Effects of Chemotherapeutic Drugs

Nadir Drug	WBC Recovery (Days)	WBC (Days)	Platelet Nadir (Days)	Comment
Asparaginase	NA[a]	NA	NA	Myelosuppression is rarely a problem
Bleomycin	NS[b]	NS	NS	NS
Busulfan	11–30	24–54	NA	
Carmustine	35–25	42–56	28–35	Cumulative delayed, prolonged myelosuppression
Chlorambucil	7–14	NA	7–14	
Cisplatin	7–10	NA	7–10	
Cyclophosphamide	8–14	18–25	10–25	Platelet-sparing
Cytarabine	12–14	22–24	22–24	Somewhat platelet-sparing
Dacarbazine	14–18	NA	14–28	
Dactinomycin	15	22–25	10–14	

Daunorubicin	10–14	21	10–14	Profound myelosuppression
Doxorubicin	14	22–54	14	
Fluorouracil	7–14	20–30	7–17	May spare platelets
Hydroxyurea	2–10	NA	NA	
Lomustine	40–50	60	28	Cumulative delayed, prolonged myelosuppression
Mechlorethamine	7–15	14–28	10–14	
Melphalan	10–12	NA	7–14	
Mercaptopurine	7	14–21	5–12	
Methotrexate	7–14	14–21	5–12	
Mitomycin	21–25	28–42	30	Cumulative prolonged myelosuppression
Mitotane	NA	NA	NA	Myelosuppression is rarely dose-limiting
Plicamycin	NA	NA	NA	Myelosuppression not usually dose-limiting

Table 5.1 (continued)

Nadir Drug	WBC Recovery (Days)	WBC (Days)	Platelet Nadir (Days)	Comment
Procarbazine	25–36	35–50+	28	Prolonged, delayed myelosuppression
Streptozocin	NA	NA	NA	Myelosuppression not usually dose-limiting
Thioguanine	8–12	NA	8–12	
Thiotepa	14–28	NA	14–28	
Vinblastine	5–9	14–21	4–10	Somewhat platelet-sparing
Vincristine	3–5	7	NA	Platelet-sparing

Source: Yancy, R. (1980). Complications of cancer chemotherapy. *Ca Bull., 32,* 168–173. (Copyright Medical Arts Publishing Foundation, Houson, Texas. Reprinted with permission.)
[a]NA = Not applicable
[b]NS = Not significant

Metabolic Alterations

Hypomagnesemia

Patients at Risk

- Receiving Carboplatin, Platinol
- Receiving long-term diuretic therapy
- With persistent nausea and vomiting
- With enterostomal drainage

Assessment

- Disorientation, confusion
- Tremors
- Cardiac dysrhythmias
- Hyperactive reflexes
- Pertinent lab values: magnesium level (normal = 1.5 mcg/liter–2.5 mcg/liter), ECG

Possible Nursing Diagnoses

- Alteration in thought processes
- Alteration in cardiac output: decreased

Nursing Actions

- Administer supplemental magnesium sulfate ($MgSO_4$ 1.0 gm IV/IM every 12 hours).
- Assess mental status at least every 8 hours; provide safety measures if patient confused.
- Monitor apical pulse rate every 4 hours.
- If tremors are severe, assist with activities of daily living.

(continued)

Metabolic Alterations (continued)

- If patient on digitalis, consult MD regarding a dose alteration. (Hypomagnesemia can potentiate effects of digitalis.)

Patient Teaching

- List signs and symptoms of hypomagnesemia.

Hyponatremia

Patients at Risk

- Receiving Carboplatin, Cyclophosphamide, Vincristine
- With persistent vomiting
- With small cell lung cancer
- On prolonged gastric suctioning

Assessment

- Change in mental status
- Lethargy
- Diarrhea
- Anorexia
- Seizure activity
- Nausea
- Pertinent lab values: sodium level (normal = 136–145 mcg/liter)

Possible Nursing Diagnoses

- Fluid volume deficit
- Potential for injury

Nursing Actions

- If Na is greater than 110 mEq/liter:
  - restrict fluids,
  - give demeclocycline 150–300 mg PO 4 times a day.
- If Na is less than 110 mEq/liter:
  - administer IV of 1 liter 3% saline or normal saline every 6 hours,
  - give furosemide (Lasix) 40–80 mg IV push every 6–8 hours,
  - monitor patient frequently for signs of fluid overload.
- Institute safety measures (siderails), if patient is confused.

Patient Teaching

- List signs and symptoms of hyponatremia.

Hypercalcemia

Patients at Risk

- With decreased mobility, bone metastasis
- With primary bone tumors, squamous cell cancer of the lung, cancer of the breast, multiple myeloma
- Receiving hormonal therapy
- Who are dehydrated

Assessment

- Nausea, vomiting
- Diarrhea, constipation

(continued)

Metabolic Alterations (continued)

- Lethargy
- Confusion
- Anorexia
- Muscle fatigue
- Hypertension
- Nocturia/polyuria
- Ataxia
- Dysrhythmias
- ECG changes (shorter Q-T interval, widening of T-wave, increased PR interval)
- Pertinent lab values: calcium (normal = 9–11 mg/100 mg or 4.5–5.5 mcg/liter), BUN, creatinine, glucose if on steroids, CBC if on mithramycin, albumin (if albumin is low, the calcium level may be higher than reported)

Possible Nursing Diagnoses

- Alteration in thought processes
- Fluid volume deficit
- Alteration in bowel elimination: constipation

Nursing Actions

- Hydrate patient with normal saline, usually 4–6 liters over 24 hours.
- Monitor intake and output closely; monitor central venous pressure in patients at risk for cardiac problems.
- Assess mental status at least every 4 hours; institute safety precautions if confused.

- Provide symptomatic relief for constipation, nausea and vomiting.
- Encourage mobility as tolerated; caution regarding increased risk for pathologic fractures.
- Monitor cardiac status as ordered.
- Review medications (Digitalis, antihypertensives, thiazide diuretics, lithium carbonate, and vitamin D may potentiate hypercalcemia.)
- Assess level of pain and medicate accordingly.
- Administer as ordered:
  - furosemide (Lasix): 40 mg IV push every 6 hours until urine output is greater than or equal to 50 cc/hour
  - mithramycin: 12.5–25 mcg/kg daily for 4–5 days
  - inorganic phosphates: 1.5–3.0 gm/day
  - steroids: 300–400 mg/day
  - calcitonin: 200–300 MRC units IM/SQ every 6–12 hours
  - prostaglandin inhibitors
  - Pamidronate Disodium (Aredia): 60–90 mg/day

Patient Teaching
- List signs and symptoms of hypercalcemia.
- Increase fluid intake to 3 liters/day.
- Increase mobility as able.
- Monitor for constipation.

(continued)

Metabolic Alterations (continued)

Hyperuricemia

Patients at Risk

- Those receiving any drug that can cause rapid tumor lysis syndrome; usually seen with lymphoma, leukemia, or multiple myeloma

Assessment

- Decrease urine output
- Hypertension
- Tachypnea
- Lethargy
- Pruritus
- Anorexia
- Diarrhea
- Edema
- Pertinent lab values: uric acid level (normal: male = 2.5–8.0 mg/100, female = 1.5–6.0 mg/100)

Possible Nursing Diagnosis

- Alteration in patterns of urinary elimination

Nursing Actions

- Administer allopurinol 200–600 mg/day; begin 24 hours prior to the initiation of chemotherapy.
- Monitor intake/output.

- Maintain alkaline urine (pH 7.0–7.5) with NAHCO$_3$.
- Force fluids to 3 liters/day.

Patient Teaching
- List signs and symptoms of hyperuricemia.
- Increase fluid intake to 3 liters/day.
- Reinforce the importance of taking allopurinol.

Nausea and Vomiting

Patients at Risk

- Receiving any chemotherapeutic agent
- Receiving radiation therapy to the abdominal region or thoracic/lumbar/sacral spine
- Taking other drugs with high emetogenic properties (e.g., analgesics, antibiotics).

Assessment

- Presence of emesis
  - frequency
  - severity
  - predisposing factors
- Baseline nutritional status
  - weight gain/loss
  - dietary habits (preparation/storage/likes/dislikes)
  - response to food
  - sociocultural influences
- Weight loss/muscle wasting
- Pertinent lab values: electrolytes, albumin, total protein

Possible Nursing Diagnoses

- Alteration in nutrition: less than body requirements
- Fluid volume deficit

Nursing Actions
- Evaluate what has been helpful in past to relieve nausea and vomiting.
- Assess for other possible causes of nausea and vomiting (e.g., obstruction, constipation, pain, other medications, psychogenic factors).
- Administer antiemetics before, during, and/or after chemotherapy administration. Note that delayed nausea and vomiting, up to 72 hours, can occur with some chemotherapy drugs (e.g., platinol, doxorubicin); refer to chapter 6.
- Administer antiemetics 30 minutes before meals.
- Choose appropriate route for antimetics (e.g., if patient is vomiting, parenteral or rectal route is preferred over oral route).
- Monitor intake and output.
- Encourage adequate fluid intake.
- Provide good oral hygiene after each emesis and before meals.
- Encourage adequate nutritional intake; provide nutritional supplements as needed.

Patient Teaching
- Eat smaller, more frequent meals and snacks.
- Take antiemetics 30 minutes prior to meals.

(continued)

Nausea and Vomiting (continued)

- Allow sufficient time for meals with rest periods.
- Avoid spicy or greasy foods.
- Take analgesics as ordered.
- Monitor self for constipation.
- Perform oral hygiene before/after meals.
- Tell family to avoid coaxing, bribing, or threatening patient in relation to food.
- Consider alternate therapies (e.g., relaxation, hypnosis, biofeedback, diversional therapy) if antiemetic therapy fails.

Neurotoxicity

Patients at Risk

- Receiving Asparaginase, Bleomycin, Cytosine Arabinoside (especially high dose), Etoposide, 5-Fluorouracil, Hydroxyurea, Ifosfamide, Mechlorethamine, Methotrexate (especially intrathecal), Paclitaxel, Platinol, Procarbazine, Vinblastine, Vincristine
- With long-term narcotic usage, spinal cord compression, uncontrolled diabetes

Assessment

- Change in mental status
- Decreased tendon reflexes
- Myalgia
- Paresthesias
- Change in bowel/bladder habits
- Gait disturbances
- Impotence
- Seizure activity
- Depression

Possible Nursing Diagnoses

- Altered thought processes
- Sensory-perceptual alteration: tactile
- Impaired physical mobility
- Alteration in bowel elimination: constipation
- Potential for injury
- Sexual dysfunction

(continued)

Neurotoxicity (continued)

Nursing Actions

- Assess cause and extent of neurotoxicities.
- Hold chemotherapy (dependent on severity of toxicity).
- Institute bowel regime for constipation; refer to Constipation, pages 176–177.
- Provide range-of-motion to extremities at least every 8 hours.
- Provide footboard/splints for footdrop.
- Inspect feet for blisters/irritation daily if peripheral neuropathies exist.
- Refer to occupational/physical therapy for use of aids (e.g., canes, walkers, safety devices).
- Institute safety precautions for changes in mental status.
- Provide pain management techniques for dysesthesias.
- Refer for sexual counseling as needed.

Patient Teaching

- List signs and symptoms of neurotoxicities.
- Stress that early detection usually leads to better resolution of the toxicity and increases chances of restoration of function.
- Instruct in the use of ambulation aids if indicated.
- Instruct in foot care if peripheral neuropathies occur.

Ototoxicity

Patients at Risk
- Receiving Platinol and its derivatives

Assessment
- Vertigo
- Tinnitus
- Hearing loss
- Pertinent lab values: serial audiograms

Possible Nursing Diagnoses
- Sensory-perceptual alteration: auditory

Nursing Actions
- If hearing loss occurs, avoid drugs that may further impair patient's hearing:
  - furosemide
  - streptomycin
  - neomycin
  - gentamycin
  - kanamycin
  - amphotericin B
- Obtain a pretreatment audiogram (hearing loss may be reversible if appropriate dose modifications are made early).

Patient Teaching
- Instruct patient to monitor and report any signs and symptoms as soon as they occur.

Pulmonary Toxicity

Patients at Risk

- Receiving BCNU, Bleomycin*, Busulfan*, Carmustine, Chlorambucil, Cyclophosphamide, Melphalan, Mercaptopurine, Methotrexate, Mitomycin*, Procarbazine
- With preexisting lung disease (e.g., COPD, Tb, asthma)
- Older than 70 years of age
- Receiving previous or concomitant radiation therapy to the chest
- With a smoking history
- Who have had chronic exposure to environmental carcinogens
- Receiving more than one chemotherapeutic agent with pulmonary toxicities
- Receiving high-tension oxygen therapy
- With impaired kidney and liver function

Assessment

- Dyspnea
- Dry cough
- Tachypnea
- Rales
- Fever
- Cyanosis
- Orthopnea

---

*High incidence

- Fatigue
- Changes in pulmonary function tests (decreased diffusion capacity, total lung volume, vital capacity)
- Anorexia
- Chest X-ray showing pulmonary infiltrates
- Pertinent lab values CBC (low Hct/Hgb can cause pulmonary symptoms; low WBC can indicate pulmonary infection); arterial blood gases (decreased pO_2, respiratory alkalosis); sputum culture and sensitivity; gram stain

Possible Nursing Diagnoses
- Impaired gas exchange
- Ineffective breathing pattern

Nursing Actions
- Assess cause of pulmonary changes (e.g., during toxicity, disease progression, non-cancerous causes).
- Discontinue chemotherapeutic agent.
- Administer steriods as ordered.
- Give O_2 only if absolutely necessary and at low rate.
- Assist patient to position of comfort (usually Fowler's position).
- Provide symptom relief for
  - anxiety,
  - cough,
  - pain.

(continued)

Pulmonary Toxicity (continued)

- Consult dietician to maintain nutritional status (calorie requirements increase with increased breathing effort).
- Work with respiratory therapy to teach patient breathing techniques (e.g., pursed lip, abdominal-diaphragmatic).
- Monitor for change in mental status (confusion could indicate hypoxia).
- Monitor vital signs (increased pulse, blood pressure, usually seen with worsening of respiratory distress).
- Maintain calm environment.
- Prevent further complications (e.g., pneumonia):
  - force fluids,
  - encourage activity as tolerated,
  - give antibiotics as ordered,
  - discourage smoking.

Patient Teaching

- List signs and symptoms of pulmonary toxicity.
- Increase fluid intake.
- Stress need to moderate activities to maintain pulmonary reserve.
- Encourage patient/family to stop smoking.

Renal Toxicity

Patients at Risk

- Receiving Cyclophosphamide, Dacarbazine, Hydroxyurea, Ifosfamide, Methotrexate (high dose), Mitomycin, Platinol, Streptozocin
- Receiving other drugs that can be nephrotoxic (e.g., aminoglycoside antibiotics, amphotericin B) as they can increase nephrotoxicity when given with chemotherapy drugs listed above

Assessment

- Change in urinary output
- Dysuria
- Hematuria
- Bilateral peripheral edema
- Increased blood pressure/respiratory rate
- Increased venous distension, especially in neck
- Weight gain
- Nausea and vomiting
- Anorexia
- Back/flank pain
- Pertinent lab values: BUN, creatinine, creatinine clearance, albumin, potassium, calcium, sodium, phosphate, magnesium, uric acid

Possible Nursing Diagnoses

- Alteration in patterns of urinary elimination
- Fluid volume excess

(continued)

Renal Toxicity (continued)

Nursing Actions

- Obtain pretreatment 24-hour urine for creatinine clearance; report if abnormal.
- Ensure vigorous hydration pre- and post-treatment (depending upon patient's condition and amount of fluid); this can be administered PO or IV.
- Monitor cardiopulmonary status during hydration, especially in the elderly or patients treated with anthracyclines (e.g., doxorubicin).
- Keep accurate intake and output during treatment.
- Measure specific gravity of all voided specimens (less than or equal to 1.030 = good hydration).
- Give diuretics (e.g., furosemide, mannitol) as ordered; monitor potassium level.
- Insert a Foley catheter as indicated for patient comfort and accuracy of output.

High-Dose Methotrexate

- Give PO or IV $NaHCO_3$ to maintain alkaline urine (ph 7.0 or greater).
- Give allopurinol 200–600 mg/day to prevent hyperuricemia; begin 24 hours prior to chemotherapy.

Patient Teaching

- List signs and symptoms of renal toxicity.
- Increase fluid intake to 3 liters/day.

Reproductive Dysfunction

Patients at Risk

- Receiving any chemotherapeutic drug, especially alkylating agents
- Receiving radiation therapy to lower abdomen, pelvis, gonads
- Who had surgical procedures on reproductive organs (e.g., hysterectomy, orchiectomy, prostatectomy, oophorectomy)

Assessment

Female

- Change in menstrual cycle
- Signs and symptoms of estrogen deficiency (e.g., hot flashes, vaginal dryness, dyspareunia)

Male

- Impotence
- Sterility
- Pertinent lab values
  - Male: serum FSH, testosterone, testicular size, sperm count and morphology
  - Female: serum FSH, LH

Possible Nursing Diagnoses

- Sexual dysfunction
- Disturbance in self-concept: body image

(continued)

Reproductive Dysfunction (continued)

Nursing Actions

- Assess level of knowledge of patient/partner.
- Obtain a brief sexual history of patient/
  partner:
  - current sexual practices,
  - importance of sexual activity,
  - knowledge of the effects of the disease
    and the treatment.
- Obtain reproductive/contraceptive history
  from patient and partner, including number
  of children or the desire to procreate.
- Counsel or refer to appropriate personnel
  where indicated (e.g., psychotherapist, sex
  therapist, genetic counselor).

Patient Teaching

- Teach effects the disease and treatment will
  have on sexual function and reproductive
  ability; include long-term side effects and
  possible return of reproductive function, if
  appropriate.
- Instruct regarding salvaging gonadal function (e.g., oophoropexy: moving of the
  ovaries out of the treatment field of radiation therapy; sperm banking).
- Teach contraceptive methods and discourage pregnancy during chemotherapy.

Sexual Dysfunction

Patients at Risk

- Receiving chemotherapy
- Receiving radiation therapy
- Who have undergone surgical procedures involving reproductive organs

Assessment

- Previous sexual history
  - painful intercourse
  - decreased vaginal lubrication
  - impotence
  - decreased libido
  - sexual activity
  - reproductive history (number of children or desire to procreate)
  - impact of previous treatment on sexual activity
  - reactions/coping mechanisms of partner
  - attitudes toward sex
  - impact of the involved body part on sexuality
  - Own feelings of sexuality, biases

Possible Nursing Diagnosis

- Sexual dysfunction

(continued)

Sexual Dysfunction (continued)

Nursing Actions

- Allow patient and partner to openly discuss their perception of how disease/treatment will affect sexuality, sexual function, and self-image.
- Discuss these perceptions and how they relate to the disease and treatment.
- Refer to appropriate counseling.
- If the patient is receiving treatment that could result in vaginal fibrosis (e.g., surgery, radiation therapy), referral for a vaginal obturator may be indicated for vaginal dilation if patient will not be having regular intercourse.

Patient Teaching

- Teach signs and symptoms of vaginal infection and importance of reporting to MD.
- If decreased vaginal lubrication is a problem, use a water-based lubricant prior to intercourse to prevent trauma and discomfort.

Stomatitis

Patients at Risk

- Receiving Bleomycin*, Cytarabine, Dactino-
  mycin*, Doxorubicin*, 5-Fluorouracil*,
  Idarubicin, Methotrexate*, Mercaptopurine,
  Plicamycin, Mitomycin, Thioguanine,
  Vinblastine, Vincristine
- With poor oral hygiene
- Receiving radiation therapy to head and
  neck area
- With poor nutritional status
- With bone-marrow depression

Assessment

- Redness, swelling of oral cavity
- White patches or sores in oral cavity
- Change in salivation
- See table 5.2
- Pertinent lab values: CBC with differential,
  platelets, albumin

Possible Nursing Diagnosis

- Alteration in oral mucous membrane
- Alteration in nutrition: less than body
  requirements
- Alteration in comfort: pain

(continued)

---

*High incidence

Stomatitis (continued)

Nursing Actions

- Assess oral cavity every 4 hours with tongue blade and pen light; note color integrity of mucosa, presence/absence of sores, consistency of salivation.
- Deliver oral hygiene using $NaHCO_3$ and H_2O, soft toothbrushes or swab, and topical anesthetics every 2–4 hours if pain is present.
- Give pain medication as needed; utilize parenteral route as needed.
- Administer antifungal agents (e.g., Nystatin, Myclex troche, Ketaconazole) as ordered.
- Administer topical analgesics (Hurricane, Dyclone, viscous lidocaine, or mixture of 1 liter normal saline or sterile water, 45–120 ml Benadryl elixir, 4 gm $NaHCO_3$, and viscous lidocaine) every 1–2 hours whenever necessary for oral discomfort.
- Give a soft, bland diet high in protein and calories.
- For severe stomatitis, use an oral power spray or Water-Pik instead of a toothbrush.

Patient Teaching

- Perform oral hygiene using soft toothbrushes or swab; rinse with 1 tsp baking soda in 8 oz warm water after each meal.

- Teach how to check oral cavity twice a day for redness, pain, patches, bleeding.
- Avoid oral irritants such as alcohol, tobacco, commercial mouth rinses, and lemon glycerine swabs.
- Keep lips moist with Vaseline, K-Y jelly, aloe, vitamin E oil.
- Have dentures checked for proper fit.
- Floss teeth only when blood counts are adequate (i.e., platelets greater than 75,000 and WBC greater than 2,000 mm^3).
- Avoid foods that are spicy, too hot, or too cold.
- Soothe sore gums by sucking on tea bags (tannic acid).

Table 5.2
Physical Assessment of the Oral Cavity[a]

Category	Rating	1	2	3	4
Lips	1 2 3 4	Smooth, soft, pink, moist, intact	Slightly dry, wrinkled, reddened areas	Dry, rough, swollen, inflammatory line of demarcation	Very dry, inflamed, cracked, blistered, ulcerated and bleeding
Tongue	1 2 3 4	Smooth, firm, pink, moist, intact	Papilli prominent, particularly at base; dry, pink with reddened areas	Raised, red papilli all over tongue giving peppered appearance; very dry and swollen, coating at base	Very dry, thick, grooved and coated; tip very red and demarcated, sides blistered

	1 2 3 4			
Oral mucosa	1 2 3 4	Smooth, pink, moist, intact	Pale, slightly dry, reddened areas or white pustules	Red, dry, inflamed, edematous, ulcerated	Very red, shiny, edematous with blisters and/or ulcerations
Teeth, dentures	1 2 3 4	Shiny, no debris; well fitting	Slightly dull with slight debris; slightly loose	Dull with debris on half of visible enamel; loose with areas of irritation	Very dull, covered with debris; unable to wear due to irritation
Saliva	1 2 3 4	Thin, watery, sufficient quantity	Increase in amount	Saliva scanty, mouth dry	Saliva thick, ropy, viscid or mucid

Source: Beck, S.(1979). Oral Exam Guide in "Impact of Teaching a Systemic Protocol for Oral Care on Stomatitis," *Cancer Nurs,* **2:**192. (Reprinted with permission.)

[a]Oral Dysfunction Score—Range: 5–20; Mild dysfunction: 6–10; Moderate dysfunction: 11–15; Severe dysfunction: 16–20.

Thrombocytopenia

Patients at Risk

- Receiving any chemotherapy; delayed thrombocytopenia (6–8 weeks after drug is administered) with Hydroxyurea, Mitomycin, nitrosoureas
- Receiving radiation therapy
- With bone-marrow depression

Assessment

- Active bleeding (e.g., wounds, oral cavity, gastrointestinal tract)
- Petechiae, ecchymosis
- Guaiac-positive stool, urine, or sputum
- Change in level of consciousness
- Hypotension
- Pertinent lab values: platelet count, Hgb/Hct, WBC

Possible Nursing Diagnoses

- Potential for injury
- Fluid volume deficit

Nursing Actions

- Monitor vital signs every 4 hours; avoid rectal temperatures.
- Label chart and lab request slips "Caution: low platelets."
- Avoid invasive procedures (e.g., enemas, urinary catheters).

- Use fine-gauge needle (e.g., 23 g, 25 g) if injections are necessary.
- Apply pressure to sites of venipunctures, injections for 5 minutes.
- Avoid aspirin or aspirin-containing drugs, anticoagulants, and alcohol.
- Limit physical activity.
- Test all secretions (e.g., stool, urine, vomit, sputum) for occult blood.
- Transfuse platelets, whole blood, or packed cells as ordered; monitor for transfusion reaction.
- Apply topical thrombin to site of active bleeding as ordered.

Patient Teaching
- List signs and symptoms of thrombo-cytopenia.
- Caution to avoid invasive procedures (e.g., dental work, flossing, enemas, douching).
- Use electric razors only.
- Use soft toothbrushes or oral swabs; keep lips lubricated.
- Use stool softeners to avoid straining.
- Take steroids with milk or antacid.
- Use a humidifier if air is dry.
- Inform female patients that their menstrual flow may be heavier than usual.

Tissue Necrosis

Patients at Risk

- Receiving vesicant agents or irritants (see table 3.1)
- With poor venous access
- With previous history of problem with or sensitivity to drug

Assessment

- Complaints
  - pain
  - burning
  - swelling
- Clinical manifestations of tissue necrosis
  - erythema
  - induration
  - tenderness
  - pain
  - ulceration, tissue breakdown

Possible Nursing Diagnoses

- Impaired tissue integrity
- Alteration in comfort: pain

Nursing Actions

- Always push irritants/vesicants slowly through the side arm of a rapidly running IV; never give direct IV push.

- Tape IV site clearly so site above needle or catheter can be observed for immediate signs of infiltration/irritation.
- In the event of an extravasation, refer to chapter 3.

Patient Teaching
- Instruct to inform RN or MD immediately if any of the above signs and symptoms occur during administration.

Venous Fibrosis/Phlebitis

Patients at Risk

- Receiving Carmustine, Dacarbazine, Doxorubicin, Etoposide, Mechlorethamine, Plicamycin, Mitomycin, Vinblastine, Vincristine

Assessment

- Along venous route
  - pain
  - redness
  - swelling
  - increased temperature
  - hardness
  - perspiration

Possible Nursing Diagnoses

- Impaired tissue integrity
- Potential for injury

Nursing Actions

- Assess venous status prior to each treatment.
- Avoid venipuncture at any compromised site (e.g., redness, swelling, soreness, mastectomy side, axillary dissection side, any extremity with edema).
- Consider adding additional diluent when administering any irritating drug.

- Apply warm compresses to any inflamed area; if a vesicant was administered, evaluate further.
- Push irritants and vesicants slowly via the side arm of a rapidly running IV; never give direct IV push.
- Flush all IV lines with a minimum of 30–50 cc of normal saline after administration.
- Rotate sites of administration regularly.
- Evaluate IV site continually during administration of drugs.

Patient Teaching
- Instruct to report any pain, burning, or redness along venous route immediately.

VI

Antiemetic Therapy

Pathophysiology

Chemotherapy-associated nausea and vomiting has been identified by patients and staff as one of the most uncomfortable side effects of treatment. In addition to the discomfort, prolonged nausea and vomiting can lead to anorexia, fluid and electrolyte imbalance, weakness, and increased susceptibility to infection. Many patients report a decrease in the quality of their life. These symptoms may become so severe that patients may choose to discontinue their treatment.

Drug-related vomiting can occur due to irritation of the gastrointestinal tract or stimulation of the chemoreceptor trigger zone (CTZ) located in the brain on the floor of the fourth ventricle. The CTZ in turn activates the vomiting center in the medulla.

Chemotherapy → CTZ → vomiting center → patient vomits

Chemotherapy is not the only cause of vomiting in oncology patients. There are many physical and psychological factors that may contribute to the patient's feelings of nausea and vomiting. Narcotics, diet, disease progression, and bowel obstruction are other contributory factors that must be assessed. A classic example of psychologic variables affecting a patient is the phenomenon of anticipatory nausea and vomiting.

This occurs when a person feels nauseous and may actually vomit *prior* to the initiation of the chemotherapy. Many times just thinking about the treatment, seeing the hospital, or smelling an alcohol swab can induce these feelings.

Pharmacologic Management

Antiemetics are administered as single agents or in combination depending on the emetic potential of the chemotherapy (high emetic potential = more antiemetics needed). Antiemetics should be started prior to the administration of chemotherapy and continued on an around-the-clock schedule for at least 24 hours. The actual incidence of vomiting decreases after 12–24 hours, but nausea may persist for a few days. The nurse should make sure that patients have antiemetics and instructions for their use when discharged from the office or hospital.

Many different classes of drugs are used as antiemetics for chemotherapy. Phenothiazines (Compazine, Thorazine, Torecan, Phenergan) have a direct effect on the vomiting center in the brain. They are commonly used as single agents for the control of mild nausea or in combination with other antiemetics for more severe symptoms. Major side effects of the phenothiazines include extrapyramidal reactions, sedation, and hypotension. Since drug metabolism occurs in the liver, caution must be used in patients with hepatic disease.

Butyrophenones (Haldol, Droperidol) inhibit the central pathways for vomiting. They are not commonly prescribed for chemotherapy-related vomiting, although their activity with platinol-induced emesis has been noted. Major side effects of the butyrophenones include extra-pyramidal reactions and sedation. Most adverse effects of these medications occur with long-term use and not with intermittent usage as indicated for chemotherapy-induced nausea and vomiting.

Metoclopramide (Reglan) has a dual action. It decreases gastric and small bowel motility as well as working directly on the vomiting center. High doses of metoclopramide (2 mg/kg) have been associated with the occurrence of extra-pyramidal reactions. These can be prevented with the addition of diphenhydramine HCl (Benadryl) 25 mg PO/IM. Other side effects include diarrhea, restlessness, and sedation. If extrapyramidal reactions occur, Benadryl 25 mg IM will reverse them.

Cannabinoids (Marinol, THC) have some effect in controlling nausea and vomiting, but the exact mechanism is not known. The main side effects include sedation, dry mouth, euphoria, and vertigo. Due to the possibility of sensory-perceptual alterations, cannabinoids should not be used in patients with psychologic problems.

Corticosteroids (Decadron) have some effect in chemotherapy-induced nausea and vomiting but the exact mechanism of action is not known. They are usually used as part of a combination antiemetic protocol.

Benzodiazepines (Lorazepam [Ativan], Diazepam [Valium]) have been administered for the control of both anticipatory and chemotherapy-induced nausea and vomiting. Ativan has been very effective in the control of patinol-induced vomiting. For controlling anticipatory nausea and vomiting, the antiemetic must be started prior to the administration of the chemotherapy. Side effects are similar to other sedatives and include sedation, disorientation, and amnesia. Side effects increase as the dosage increases and the nurse must closely monitor the patient for possible oversedation and aspiration.

Ondansetron-Hydrochloride (Zofran) and Granisetron (Kytril) act as blocking agents to serotonin. Their greatest efficacy is at the time of chemotherapy administration rather than as maintenance therapy. Their side effects are minimal and include headache, constipation, and transient elevation of liver chemistries.

Nausea and vomiting can usually be controlled or minimized with careful patient assessment and judicious use of combination antiemetic therapy adjusted to meet the individual patient's needs.

Examples of Antiemetic Protocols
Example 1

Ativan 2 mg PO	
Benadryl 50 mg PO	30 minutes before
Compazine 10 mg PO	chemo
Decadron 20 mg IV	

Compazine 10 mg PO/IM	Every 4 hours prn

Example 2

Ativan 1–2 mg IV/PO	30 min before chemo, then every 6 hours × 3 doses
Reglan 2 mg/kg IV	30 min before chemo and 1½, 3½, 5½ hours after chemo
Benadryl 25–50 mg PO/IV	30 min before chemo, then every 6 hours × 3 doses
Decadron 4–12 mg IVPB	30 min before chemo, then every 6 hours × 3 doses

Example 3

Decadron 20 mg IV	Before chemo
Ondansetron 32 mg IV bolus	Before chemo

For patients managing delayed nausea and vomiting:

Metoclopramide 0.5 mg/kg PO	QID × 4 days
Decadron 4–8 mg PO	BID × 4 days
Ondansetron 8 mg PO	TID × 2–5 days

Nonpharmacologic Management

The intimate relationship between mind and body with respect to nausea and vomiting cannot be underestimated. This has been clearly demonstrated with anticipatory nausea and vomiting. Based on this relationship, non-pharmacologic methods of antiemetic therapy have been developed and are being utilized on a more frequent basis.

While many patients will have a good response to combination antiemetic drug therapy, there remains a cohort of patients for whom nausea and vomiting remains a problem both pre- and post-chemotherapy. Previous experience with chemotherapy-induced emesis as well as a high level of anxiety appear to be significant contributory factors in this intractable nausea and vomiting.

Techniques such as relaxation, diversion therapy, biofeedback, and hypnosis have all been utilized with varying degrees of success. These techniques can be employed by most patients and are usually used in conjunction with a pharmacologic antiemetic regimen.

Relaxation techniques such as progressive muscle tension-relaxation, controlled breathing, and guided imagery can be taught by the nurse and practiced by the patient. Guided imagery is simply a technique used to take the person mentally out of their current situation by using their imagination to create a relaxing scene, story, or mood.

An easy technique for progressive muscle tension-relaxation is as follows:

- Find a calm/quiet environment.
- Get in a comfortable position.
- Close your eyes.
- Take a deep breath in through your nose.
- Count to 5 and let the breath out slowly through your mouth; repeat × 2.
- Now, in order, tighten your forehead, eyelids, cheeks, chin, jaw, neck, shoulders, upper arms, forearms, fist, buttocks, thighs, calves, feet, and toes; hold each for 3 counts and relax.
- Remain still for a while; concentrate on your breathing; listen to the quiet.

- Take a deep breath in through your nose.
- Count to 5 and breathe out slowly through your mouth.
- Open your eyes.

Biofeedback and hypnosis require the intervention of a specially trained person (e.g., therapist, psychiatrist, psychologist). Biofeedback also requires the use of electronic equipment for response feedback. With training and practice, however, many patients can become self-directed in these techniques.

Diversion therapy may include the use of music, reading, TV, crafts, or anything that rechannels the patient's focus away from the thoughts of nausea and vomiting.

It is important to remember that just as patients' response to chemotherapy are individualized, so too are their responses to antimetic therapy. It is a vital component of the nurse's role to assess the patient's antiemetic needs and implement appropriate pharmacologic and nonpharmacologic measures to meet these needs.

Table 6.1
Frequently Used Antiemetics

Drug	Route	Dose	Frequency
Chlorpromazine (Thorazine)	IM/IV PO Rectal	12.5–50 mg 10–50 mg 50–100 mg	q3–4h q4–6h q6–8h
Delta-9-tetrahydro-cannabinol (Marinol)	PO	2.5–10 mg	q2–4h up to 6 doses/day
Dexamethasone (Decadron)	IM/IV PO	8–20 mg 10–40 mg	q4–6h q3–4h
Diphenhydramine HCl (Benadryl)	IM/IV PO	25–50 mg 25–50 mg	q6h q6h
Granisetron (Kytril)	IV	32 mg	30 min prechemo
Haloperidol (Haldol)	IM/IV PO	2–4 mg	q6–8h
Hydroxyzine (Atarax, Vistaril)	IM PO	25–100 mg	q4–6h
Inapsine (Droperidol)	IV/IM	1.25 mg 2.5 mg	q4–6h

Drug	Route	Dose	Frequency
Lorazepam (Ativan)	IM/IV	0.5–3 mg	q6–8h
	PO		q4–6h
Metoclopramide (Reglan)	IV	1–2 mg/kg	Varies greatly (see individual protocols)
	PO	10 mg	
Ondansetron HCl (Zofran)	IV	0.15 mg/kg	30 min prechemo
			4 hrs postchemo
			8 hrs postchemo
	PO	32 mg	30 min prechemo
		8 mg	Every 8 hrs postchemo × 72 hrs
Prochlorperazine (Compazine)	IM/IV	10 mg	q4h
	PO	10–20 mg	q4h
	Rectal	25 mg	q4h
Promethazine (Phenergan)	IM/IV	12.5–25 mg	q4–6h
	PO	25 mg	
	Rectal	25 mg	
Thiethylperazine (Torecan)	IM	10 mg	TID
	PO	10–20 mg	
	Rectal	10 mg	
Trimethobensamide (Tigan)	IM	200 mg	TID
	PO	250 mg	
	Rectal	200 mg	

VII

Safe Handling of Chemotherapeutic Agents

Concern regarding potential hazards to health care workers who handle cytotoxic agents has grown over the past several years. Many of these agents are known to be mutagenic or carcinogenic. However, no conclusive research has shown them to be hazardous to the people who mix and administer them. One thing that has been shown is the exposure potential, and traditional drug handling techniques do not offer sufficient protection.

The following guidelines are recommended when working with chemotherapeutic agents.

General Guidelines

1. Only personnel trained in the mixing and administration of chemotherapy should be allowed to do so.
2. The mixing and administration of chemotherapy should take place in a quiet environment. Smoking, eating, and drinking should be banned from this area.
3. All IV syringes and tubing connections should have Luer-Lok fittings.
4. Needles should never be clipped since this increases chance of generating drug aerosols.
5. All syringes, IV bottles and bags must be labeled with the patient's name and room number, drug name, dosage, route of administration, date and time of preparation, and expiration date.

6. Always wash hands before and after working with chemotherapy.
7. Pregnant personnel should not mix chemotherapy. It is the individual institution's responsibility to develop policies regarding the administration of chemotherapy by pregnant personnel and the follow-up care of chemotherapy patients when the handling of waste products is involved.

Mixing

1. Use a Biologic Safety Cabinet (laminar airflow hood is the most common).
2. Wear 2 pairs of latex gloves (change every hour).
3. Wear a protective gown with long sleeves and closed knit cuffs.
4. Use an aerosol micro-pore filter to equalize pressure in the drug vials and prevent spray-back of the drug.
5. Goggles are optional, but are advised when mixing chemotherapy outside a Biologic Safety Cabinet.
6. Never expel air from a syringe into room air as it may contain drug residue. Use an empty vial to expel air and/or excess drug. Dispose of this vial as biohazardous waste.
7. Wrap sterile gauze around needles and vial tops when withdrawing solution.

8. Exercise particular caution with respect to needle sticks.

Administration

1. Wear latex gloves and protective gown with long sleeves and closed knit cuffs.
2. Mask and goggles are optional.
3. Check the fitting of IV tubing and syringes carefully.
4. Prime tubing with a 50-cc flush bag of D_5W or normal saline if possible. If not, prime tubing into a sterile gauze pad in a plastic bag; dispose of as biohazardous waste.
5. Needleless systems are recommended to prevent accidental needle sticks.

Disposal

1. Personnel handling waste products (e.g., vomit, urine, blood) from patients who have received chemotherapy within 48 hours should wear gloves and protective gowns.
2. Dispose of all equipment (e.g., syringes, needles, IV tubing, bottles, bags) according to institution policy for biohazardous waste materials.
3. Place needles, syringes, and breakable items in a puncture-proof container marked biohazardous waste.

4. Ensure that a specially designated container for disposal of chemotherapy equipment is available in every area where the drugs are prepared or administered.

Spills

1. Use a commercially prepared spill kit; follow manufacturer directions.
2. *Spills of less than 5 cc* are to be cleaned immediately by trained personnel wearing double latex gloves, gowns, and goggles.
3. Ensure that absorbent gauze pads or plastic-backed absorbent paper is used to wipe the area, followed by a thorough cleansing with a detergent.
4. Cover *spills larger than 5 cc* with an absorbent pad. Personnel should wear double latex gloves, protective gown, goggles, and respirator (available in spill kit). After spill is absorbed into pad, clean the area with a detergent solution followed by rinsing with water. Dispose of all materials in receptacles labeled biohazardous waste.

More in-depth guidelines are available from the Occupational Safety and Health Administration, National Cancer Institute, or the American Cancer Society.

Appendices

Appendix I
Blood Parameters

(Normal blood values may vary slightly with different laboratories.)

CBC with Differential

Hematocrit	Men: 47% (40%–54%)
	Women: 42% (37%–47%)
Hemoglobin	Men: 14–18 gm
	Women: 12–16 gm
	Children: 12–14 gm
Erthrocytes	Men: (4.5–6) × 10^6 mm^3
	Women: 4.3–5.5 × 10^6 mm^3
Reticulocytes	Men: 0.8%–2.5%
	Women: 0.8%–4.1%
Leukocytes, total	5,000–10,000 mm^3 100%
Segmented neutrophils	1,800–6,500 mm^3 40%–60%
Lymphocytes	1,000–4,000 mm^3 20%–40%
Monocytes	200–800 mm^3 4%–8%
Band neutrophils	0–700 mm^3 3%
Eosinophils	50–400 mm^3 1%–3%
Basophils	0–150 mm^3 0%–1%
Myelocytes	-0- 0%
Platelets	150,000–350,000 mm^3

Blood Chemistries

Albumin	3.5–5.5 gm/100 cc
Ammonia	40–70 mcg/100 cc

Billirubin
   Direct   0.1–0.4 mg/100 cc
   Indirect   0.2–0.7 mg/100 cc
   Total   0.3–1.1 mg/100 cc
BUN   10–20 mg/100 cc
Calcium   4.5–5.5 mEq/liter
                    9–11 mg/100 cc
Chloride   100–106 mEq/liter
                    355–376 mg/100 cc as Cl
                    585–620 mg/100 cc as NaCl
Cholesterol   150–250 mg/100 cc
Creatinine (serum)   0.7–1.5 mg/100 cc
Fibrinogen, plasma   200–400 mg/100 cc
Folic acid   6–15 mg/cc
Glucose (fasting)   70–105 mg/100 cc
Immunoglobulins
   IgA   90–325 mg/100 cc
   IgG   800–1,500 mg/100 cc
   IgM   45–150 mg/100 cc
Iron   75–175 mcg/100 cc
Iron binding capacity 150–300 mcg/100 cc
Lactic acid   6–16 mg/100 cc
Lipids (total)   450–850 mg/100 cc
Magnesium   1.5–2.5 mEq/liter
                    1.8–3 mg/100 cc
Phosphate, inorganic   3–4.5 mg/100 cc
Potassium   3.5–5 mEq/liter
Protein (total)   6–8 gm/100 cc
Sodium   136–145 mEq/liter

(continued)

Blood Parameters (continued)

Uric acid
    Males   2.5–8.0 mg/100 cc
    Females   1.5–6.0 mg/100 cc

Arterial Blood Gases
pH   7.35–7.45
pO_2 80–100 mmHg
pCO_3 35–45 mmHg
HCO_3 22–26 mEq/liter
O_2 saturation   95% or greater
Base excess   −2 to +2

Appendix II
Nomograms for Determining Body Surface Area (M²)

Infants and Young Children, page 254
Older Children and Adults, page 255

To determine the surface area of the patient, draw a straight line between the point representing his/her height on the left vertical scale to the point representing his/her weight on the right vertical scale. The point at which this line intersects the middle vertical scale represents the surface area in square meters. (Courtesy of Abbott Laboratories)

Alternate Method
The following formula can be used to calculate the body surface area for older children and adults:

$$\sqrt{\frac{\text{Height (in inches)} \times \text{weight (in pounds)}}{3131}}$$

Nomograms for Body Surface Area

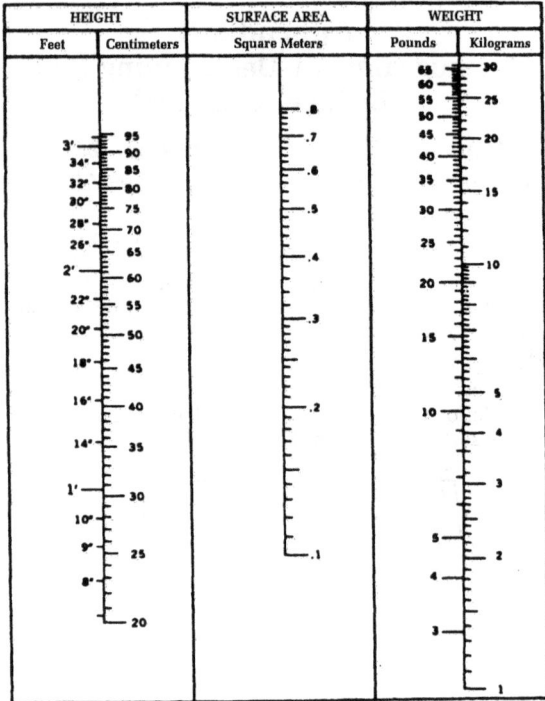

HEIGHT		SURFACE AREA	WEIGHT	
Feet	Centimeters	Square Meters	Pounds	Kilograms

Source: Courtesy of Abbott Laboratories.

Memory Bank for Chemotherapy

HEIGHT		SURFACE AREA	WEIGHT	
Feet	Centimeters	Square Meters	Pounds	Kilograms

		3.00	440	200
	220	2.90	420	190
7'	215	2.80	400	180
10"	210	2.70	380	170
8"	205	2.60	360	160
6"	200	2.50	340	150
4"	195	2.40	320	140
2"	190	2.30	300	
6'	185	2.20	290 280	130
10"	180	2.10	270 260	120
8"	175	2.00	250 240	110
6"	170	1.95 1.90	230	
4"	165	1.85	220	100
2"	160	1.80	210	95
5'	155	1.75 1.70	200	90
10"	150	1.65	190	85
8"	145	1.60	180	80
6"	140	1.55 1.50	170	75
4"	135	1.45 1.40	160	70
2"	130	1.35	150	65
4'	125	1.30	140	60
10"	120	1.25	130	55
8"	115	1.20 1.15	120	50
6"	110	1.10 1.05	110	45
4"	105	1.00	100	40
2"	100	.95	90	35
3'	95	.90	80	30
10"	90	.85	70	25
8"	85	.80	60	20
6"	80	.75 .70	50	
	75	.65 .60		

Appendix III
Patient Assessment Form

Name _____

Address _____

_____

Telephone _____ Date of Birth _____

Hospital Number _____ Allergies _____

Employment _____

Insurance _____

Significant Other _____

   Address & Phone Number _____

Past Medical History

Illnesses	Dates	Treatments
_____	_____	_____
_____	_____	_____
_____	_____	_____

Surgery

_____	_____	_____
_____	_____	_____

Medications	Dosage	Last taken
_____	_____	_____
_____	_____	_____
_____	_____	_____
_____	_____	_____

Chemotherapy	Date	Reaction
_____	_____	_____
_____	_____	_____

Radiation Therapy

_____ _____ _____
_____ _____ _____

Current Medical Situation
Diagnosis   Date   Stage/Site

_____ _____ _____
Metastasis _____
Proposed treatment _____
Tests _____
_____
Is chemotherapy investigational? _____
Signed consent on chart? _____

Patient Knowledge of Disease and Treatment
Knows diagnosis _____
States names of drugs _____
States side effects of drugs and how to manage them
_____
Has written materials on drugs/disease _____
Needs further education regarding disease and
treatment _____
COMMENTS _____
_____

Support Systems/Resources
Family _____
Financial _____
Home care _____
Housing _____
Transportation _____
Counseling _____
Refer to _____
COMMENTS _____

(continued)

Patient Assessment Form (continued)

Review Lab Data

RBC _____ HGB _____ HCT _____

WBC _____

    Neutrophils _____

    Lymphocytes _____

    Monocytes _____

    Bands _____

Platelets _____

Date of last chest X-ray _____

Date of last cardiac ejection fraction scan (MUGA)

_____

    Normal _____ Abnormal _____ Result _____ % _____

T: _____ P: _____ R: _____ BP: _____

Height: _____ Weight: _____ BSA _____ /M²

    Weight loss or gain _____

Other scans: Bone: _____

             Liver/Spleen: _____

             Other: _____

Vascular Access

Right atrial catheter _____ Site _____ Date _____

Implantable port _____ Site _____ Date _____

Implantable pump _____ Site _____ Date _____

Is patient capable of self-care regarding vascular

access device? _____

    If no, who cares for device? _____

    Is further instruction necessary? _____

COMMENTS _____

_____

_____

Systems Review

Cardiovascular
Cumulative dosage of Anthracycline _____/M²
Risks: History of cardiac disease _____
       Past or concurrent radiation to mediastinal area

_____

Signs and Symptoms of CHF
    SOB _____ Rales _____ Edema _____ Cyanosis _____
    Dizziness _____ Pulse (apical) _____ Regular _____
                                            Irregular _____
ECG (result and date) _____
MUGA (result and date) _____
Venous distension (site) _____
Venous fibrosis (site) _____

Gastrointestinal
Anorexia _____ No. of meals/day _____ Best meal _____
Food aversions _____
Food likes _____
Nausea/vomiting _____ Medication _____
    Effective _____
    Other treatments for nausea/vomiting _____
    Effective _____
Constipation _____ Medication _____
    Effective _____
    Other treatments for constipation _____
    Effective _____
Diarrhea _____ Frequency _____ Medication _____
    Effective _____
    Other treatments for diarrhea _____
    Effective _____

(continued)

Patient Assessment Form (continued)

Ostomy _____ Type _____ Self-care _____
 Refer to enterostomal therapist _____
Mucositis _____ Describe _____

 _____

 Current oral care _____

 _____

 Instructed in oral care _____

 _____

 Medications for mucositis _____
 Effective _____
 Other treatments for mucositis _____
 Effective _____
 Dentures _____ Proper fit _____
Abdominal fullness/tenderness _____ Site _____
Jaundice _____

Hematologic

Skin color _____
Energy level (0 = bedbound; 5 = able to carry out
ADL without problems) _____
Dizziness _____
Fever _____
C&S: Urine _____ Sputum _____ Blood _____
 Catheter _____ Wound _____
Abnormal discharge _____ Site _____
Bruising _____ Site _____
Bleeding _____ Site _____
Allergies _____ Site _____
Menses _____ Last menstrual period _____

Integumentary

Skin turgor _____

Alopecia _____ Wig _____ Referral _____

Venous route discoloration _____

Rash _____ Site _____

Allergies _____

Nervous

Paresthesias _____ Site _____

Change in gait _____

Change in bowel/bladder habits _____

Hearing loss _____

Ataxia _____ Dizziness _____

Prior treatment with vinca alkaloids or platinum _____

Genitourinary

Urinary pattern

    Pain _____ Frequency _____ Urgency _____

    Odor _____ Blood _____

History of urinary tract infections _____

    Dates _____ Treatments _____

Ostomy _____ Type _____ Self-care _____

    Refer to enterostomal therapist _____

Sexual/Reproductive Function

Is patient sexually active? _____

Does patient practice birth control? _____ Type _____

Is patient/partner encountering problems regarding

    sexual reproductive function? _____

    Pain _____ Impotence _____

    Vaginal dryness _____

    Decreased libido _____ Infertility _____

    Other _____

(continued)

Patient Assessment Form (continued)

Does patient/partner have desire for children? _____

Is patient aware of drug effects on sexual/reproductive
   function? _____

Refer for counseling _____

Refer for sperm banking _____

Respiratory

Chest X-ray (result and date) _____

Pulmonary function test (result and date) _____

Cough _____ Productive _____ Sputum C&S _____

Risks: Cumulative dose of Bleomycin _____/M^2

   History of pulmonary disease _____

   Past or concurrent radiation to chest _____

   History of smoking (years) _____

   Packs/day _____

Orthopnea _____ Number of pillows _____

Any history of allergic reaction to medicines _____

_____
_____

Nurse's Name _____ Date _____

Appendix IV
Chemotherapy Checklist

Before Administration of Any Drug
_____ Right patient (assures patient identification)
_____ Right drug (correctly labeled)
_____ Right route
_____ Right time
_____ Right dose
_____ Inform patient of drug being administered
_____ Is patient alert, oriented?
_____ If drug is investigational, is proper consent
signed?

Neurologic (CNS) Assessment
_____ Is drug neurotoxic?
_____ Is patient aware?
_____ Are any neurotoxicites present (numbness,
tingling, gait disturbance, mental changes)?
_____ Is physician aware of any neurotoxicities that
are present?
_____ Has patient been taught how to manage neuro
side effects?

Cardiac Assessment
_____ Is drug cardiotoxic?
_____ Is patient aware?

(continued)

Chemotherapy Checklist (continued)

_____ Are any cardiac toxicities present (abnormal cardiac ejection fraction, abnormal rhythm)?
_____ Is physician aware of an abnormal cardiac side effects?
_____ Has patient been taught to manage cardiac side effects?

Gastrointestinal Assessment
_____ Have antiemetics been ordered?
_____ Dose drug cause gastrointestinal side effects (e.g., diarrhea, constipation, nausea/vomiting, stomatitis)?
_____ Is patient aware?
_____ Has patient been taught how to manage symptoms (e.g., informed on antiemetics, antidiarrhea)?
_____ Has oral hygiene practice been established?

Hematologic Assessment
_____ Does patient have normal CBC (WBC, Hgb, platelets)?
_____ If not, is physician aware?

Pulmonary Assessment
_____ Does drug being given cause pulmonary toxicities?
_____ Is patient aware?
_____ Are any pulmonary toxicities present (normal pulmonary function tests, regular respiration)?

_____ Is physician aware of any abnormal pulmonary symptoms?
_____ Is patient receiving radiation therapy to chest area?

Genitourinary Assessment
_____ Does drug have any genitourinary side effects?
_____ Is patient aware?
_____ Are any genitourinary side effects present (e.g., proteinuria; increased BUN, creatinine or creatinine clearance)?

Integumentary Assessment
_____ Are skin and orifices intact (e.g., no symptoms of infection, hemorrhage, rash)?
_____ Does drug cause alopecia?
_____ Is patient aware?
_____ Is physician aware of any symptoms?
_____ Has patient been taught to manage side effects?
_____ Does patient have a wig or toupee?

Hepatic Assessment
_____ Does drug cause hepatotoxicities?
_____ Is patient aware?
_____ Are any hepatic toxicities present (e.g., increased alkaline phosphatase, LDH, SGOT, SGPT; palpable liver, jaundice)?
_____ Is physician aware of any symptoms?

(continued)

Chemotherapy Checklist (continued)

Reproductive/Sexual Function Assessment

____ Does drug cause alterations in reproductive function?

____ Does drug cause alterations in libido or sexual function?

____ Is patient aware of these potential dysfunctions?

____ Is counseling available to the patient?

Intravenous Status

____ Is appropriate IV access device in use (e.g., butterfly, angiocath, right atrial catheter)?

____ Is there a good blood return?

____ Is site without redness or swelling?

____ Is IV fluid free flowing?

____ Is IV fluid compatible with drugs?

Appendix V
Postchemotherapy Administration
Checklist

_____ Does patient understand potential side effects
      and how to prevent/minimize them?
_____ Has patient received instructions on
      antiemetics, diet, follow-up appointments (e.g.,
      lab or physician)?
_____ Have appropriate referrals been made to
      American Cancer Society, Social Service, Home
      Care (e.g., counseling, wigs)?
_____ Does patient have appropriate phone numbers
      (e.g., physician, nurse, clinic, social worker)?
_____ Is phone follow-up necessary?

Bibliography

Anderson R, Puckett W: *Establishing an Oncology Pharmacy Service*. Syracuse, NY, Bristol Myers, 1987.

Barton Burke M, Wilkes G, Berg D, Bean C, and Ingluersen K: *Cancer Chemotherapy A Nursing Process Approach*. Boston, Jones & Bartlett Publishers, 1991.

Beck S: Impact of a systematic oral care protocol on stomatitis after chemotherapy. *Cancer Nurs* 2:185–199, 1979.

Brandt B: A nursing protocol for the client with neutropenia. *Oncol Nurs Forum* 11:24–28, 1984.

Cancer: Chemotherapy and Care (Parts I and II). Syracuse, NY, Bristol Laboratories, 1981.

Cancer chemotherapy: guidelines and recommendations for nursing education and practice. Pittsburgh, Oncology Nursing Society, 1984, 1988.

Cherneckey C, Ramsey P: *Crucial nursing care of the client with cancer*. Norwalk, CT, Appleton-Century-Crofts, 1984.

Conrad K: Cerebellar toxicities associated with cytosine arabinoside: A nursing perspective. *Oncol Nurs Forum* 13:57–59, 1986.

Cozzi E, et al: Nursing management of patients receiving hepatic arterial chemotherapy through an implanted infusion pump. *Cancer Nurs* 7:229–234, 1984.

Craig J, Capizzi R: The prevention and treatment of immediate hypersensitivity reactions from cancer chemotherapy. *Seminars Oncol Nurs* 1:285–291, 1985.

Delisa AF, Flannelly BP, Gregory RE: Administration and Use of Cancer Chemotherapeutic Agents. *Oncology Reference Manual.* New York, The McMahon Group, 1995.

Donoghue M, Nunnally J, Yasko J: *Nutritional Aspects of Cancer Care.* Reston, VA, Reston Publishing, 1982.

Door R, Fritz W: *Cancer Chemotherapy Handbook.* New York, Elsevier, 1980.

Engelking C, Steele N: A model for pretreatment nursing assessment of patients receiving cancer chemotherapy. *Cancer Nurs* 7:203–212, 1984.

Frank J: The effects of music therapy and guided visual imagery on chemotherapy-induced nausea and vomiting. *Oncol Nurs Forum* 12:47–52, 1985.

Gannon C: Bleeding due to Thrombocytopenia. In J. Yasko (ed.): *Nursing management of symptoms associated with chemotherapy.* Reston, VA, Reston Publishing, 1983.

Govoni L, Hayes J: *Drugs and Nursing Implications* (5th ed.). Norwalk, CT, Appleton-Century-Crofts, 1986.

Groenwald S (ed.): *Cancer Nursing: Principles and Practice.* Boston, Jones & Barlett Publishers, 1987.

Harder L, Hatfield A: Patient participation in monitoring myelosuppression from chemotherapy. *Oncol Nurs Forum* 9:35–37, 1982.

Ignoffo R, Friedman M: Therapy of local toxicities caused by extravasation of cancer chemotherapeutic drugs. *Cancer Treat Rev* 7:17–27, 1980.

Jassak P, Sticklin L: Interleukin-2: An overview. *Oncol Nurs Forum* 13:17–22, 1986.

Kaempfer A: The effects of cancer chemotherapy on reproduction: A review of the literature. *Oncol Nurs Forum* 8:11–18, 1981.

Kaszyk L: Cardiac toxicity associated with cancer therapy. *Oncol Nurs Forum* 13:81–88, 1986.

Knobf M: Intravenous therapy guidelines for oncology practice. *Oncol Nurs Forum* 9:30–34, 1982.

Knobf MK, Lewis KP, Fischer PS, Schneider WR, Weech D: *Cancer Chemotherapy: Treatment and Care*. Boston, G.K. Hale Publishers, 1981.

Krakoff I: Cancer chemotherapeutic agents. *CA—A Cancer J Clinicians* 31:130–140, 1981.

Kreamer K: Anaphylaxis resulting from chemotherapy. *Oncol Nurs Forum* 8:13–16, 1981.

Lauffer B, Yasko J: *Care of the Client Receiving Chemotherapy: A Self-Learning Module for the Nurse Caring for the Client with Cancer*. Reston, VA, Reston Publishers, 1984.

Maxwell M: Scalp tourniquets for chemotherapy-induced alopecia. *Am J Nurs* 80:900–903, 1980.

Maxwell M: When the cancer patient becomes anemic. *Cancer Nurs* 7:321–326, 1984.

McNally J, Stair J, Somerville E: *Guidelines for Cancer Nursing Practice*. New York, Grune & Stratton, 1985.

Oncology Nursing Society: Guidelines for nursing care of patients with altered protective mechanisms, altered hemostatis—thrombocytopenia secondary to chemotherapy. *Oncol Nurs Forum* 9:89–92, 1982.

Memory Bank for Chemotherapy

Perry MC: *The Cancer Chemotherapy Source Book.* Baltimore, MD, Williams and Wilkins, 1992.

Pinedo HM, Longo DL, Chabner BA: *Cancer Chemotherapy and Biological Response Modifiers.* Amsterdam, Elsevier Publishers, 1994.

Preston F: Management of oral bleeding caused by thrombocytopenia. *Oncol Nurs Forum* 10:59, 1983.

Trissel LA: *Handbook on Injectable Drugs* (7th ed.). Washington DC, American Society of Hospital Pharmacists, 1992.

Weiss R, Trush D: A review of pulmonary toxicity of cancer chemotherapeutic agents. *Oncol Nurs Forum* 9:16–21, 1982.

Wickham R: Pulmonary toxicity secondary to cancer treatment. *Oncol Nurs Forum* 13:69–76, 1986.

Wilkes G, Vannicola P, Steve P: Long term venous access. *Am J Nurs* 85:793–796, 1985.

Winters V: Implantable vascular access devices. *Oncol Nurs Forum* 11:25–30, 1984.

Wood H, Ellerhorst-Ryan J: Delayer adverse skin reactions associated with mitmomycin-C administration. *Oncol Nurs Forum* 11:14–18, 1984.

Yasko J (ed.): *Guidelines for Cancer Symptom Management.* Reston, VA, Reston Publishers, 1983.

Zook von Enck D: Management of Chemotherapy Induced Nausea and Vomiting: An Update. *Challenges in Treatment and Management. Proceedings of the Sixth National Conference on Cancer Nursing.* ACS, 1992.

www.ingramcontent.com/pod-product-compliance
Lightning Source LLC
Chambersburg PA
CBHW060344220326
41598CB00023B/2803